Medicine

MEDICAL EXAMINATION REVIEW

Medicine
Eighth Edition

800 Multiple Choice Questions With
Referenced Explanatory Answers

Michael A. Baker, M.D., FRCP(C), FACP
Professor of Medicine
Faculty of Medicine
University of Toronto
Ontario, Canada

MEDICAL EXAMINATION PUBLISHING CO., INC.
an Excerpta Medica company

Main entry under title:

Medical examination review.

    Vol. published in New Hyde Park, N.Y.
    Includes various editions of some volumes.
    Includes bibliographical references.
    1. Medicine—Examinations, questions, etc.
RC58.M4   610'.76   61-66847
ISBN 0-87488-102-1   AACR1

Copyright © 1984 by
MEDICAL EXAMINATION PUBLISHING CO., INC.
an Excerpta Medica company
3003 New Hyde Park Road
New Hyde Park, New York

All rights reserved. No part of this publication
may be reproduced in any form or by any means,
electronic or mechanical, including photocopy,
without permission in writing from the publisher.

Printed in the United States of America

notice

The author and the publisher of this book have made every effort to ensure that all therapeutic modalities that are recommended are in accordance with accepted standards at the time of publication.

The drugs specified within this book may not have specific approval by the Food and Drug Administration in regard to the indications and dosages that are recommended by the author. The manufacturer's package insert is the best source of current prescribing information.

Contents

Preface   vii

1. Infectious Diseases, Immunology, and Allergy   1
   Answers and Comments   23

2. Diseases of the Digestive System   33
   Answers and Comments   48

3. Diseases of the Respiratory System   56
   Answers and Comments   74

4. Diseases of the Cardiovascular System   82
   Answers and Comments   107

5. Diseases of the Blood   119
   Answers and Comments   139

6. Diseases of the Kidneys: Fluids and Electrolytes   148
   Answers and Comments   161

7. Diseases of Nutrition, Metabolism, and Endocrines   168
   Answers and Comments   191

8. Diseases of the Musculoskeletal System   203
   Answers and Comments   217

9. Diseases of the Nervous System   224
   Answers and Comments   238

vi / Contents

10. Clinical Pharmacology 245
    Answers and Comments 257

11. Diseases of the Skin 264
    Answers and Comments 272

12. Legal Medicine 277
    Answers and Comments 284

    References 288

Preface

This eighth edition of *Medical Examination Review: Volume 2, Medicine* has been substantially revised and updated to keep in step with current trends in medical education and the continuing expansion of scientific knowledge. It is designed to help you prepare for course examinations, National Boards Part II, the Federation Licensing Examination (FLEX), and examinations for foreign medical graduates.

The range of subjects included in this volume is based on the content outline of the National Board of Medical Examiners, which develops the question pool for the tests mentioned above, and reflects the scope and depth of what is taught in medical schools today. The questions themselves are organized in broad categories, to give you a representative sampling of the material covered in course work, while helping you define those general areas to which you need to devote attention. For your convenience in selective study, the answers (with commentary and references) follow each section of questions.

Each question has been scrutinized by specialists to verify that it is relevant and current. The author's care in item construction gives you questions that will provide good practice in familiarizing yourself with the format of objective-type tests. Questions of each type—one best response, matching, multiple true-false, and so on—are grouped together. They are modeled as closely as possible after those used by the Board.

Using this book, you may identify areas of strength and weakness in your own command of the subject. Specific references to widely used textbooks allow you to return to the authoritative source for further study. This volume supplements the lettered answers with brief explanations intended to prompt you to think about the choices—correct and incorrect, to put the answers in broadened perspective, and to add to your fund of knowledge. A complete bibliography appears at the end of the book. The questions and answers, taken together, emphasize problem solving and application of underlying principles as well as retention of factual knowledge.

disclaimer

The author has made every effort to thoroughly verify the answers to the questions which appear on the following pages. However, as in any text, some inaccuracies and ambiguities may occur; therefore, if in doubt, please consult your references.

The Publisher

1. Infectious Diseases, Immunology, and Allergy

DIRECTIONS: Each of the questions or incomplete statements below is followed by five suggested answers or completions. Select the **one** that is **best** in each case.

1. In coccidioidomycosis
   A. the prognosis is worse for children than for adults
   B. the great majority of infections are clinically manifest
   C. there is a greater incidence in northern than southern California
   D. there is no seasonal distribution
   E. the prognosis is worse for Negroes than Caucasians

2. Subacute sclerosing panencephalitis
   A. responds to tetracycline
   B. is usually self-limiting
   C. causes largely sensory symptoms
   D. is a late complication of measles
   E. is a late complication of scarlet fever

3. Clinical manifestations of enterovirus infections may include all of the following EXCEPT
   A. fever
   B. aseptic meningitis
   C. myalgia
   D. exanthems
   E. Horner's syndrome

4. Death from influenza is usually due to
   A. encephalitis
   B. tracheobronchitis
   C. pneumonia
   D. myocarditis
   E. adrenal collapse

5. A food poisoning epidemic resulting from ingestion of cream-filled pastry is most likely due to
   A. staphylococcal enterotoxin
   B. *Clostridium botulinum*
   C. *Clostridium perfringens*
   D. *Salmonella* species
   E. ptomaine poisoning

6. Live rubella vaccine should be given to
   A. children between one year and puberty
   B. infants less than one year
   C. all adults
   D. pregnant women
   E. all exposed patients

7. The primary manifestation of hookworm infection is
   A. bowel obstruction
   B. generalized rash
   C. anemia
   D. fever
   E. renal failure

8. The most frequent complication of measles is
   A. pneumonia
   B. encephalitis
   C. otitis media
   D. bronchitis
   E. mastoiditis

9. Granuloma inguinale is associated with all of the following clinical findings EXCEPT
   A. ulcerative skin lesions
   B. extensive scarring
   C. limitation to the inguinal area
   D. vegetative lesions
   E. response to amphotericin B

10. *Histoplasma capsulatum* may be best characterized as
    A. causing a localized infection
    B. an intracellular organism found in the reticuloendothelial (RE) system
    C. an encapsulated bacterium
    D. sensitive to large doses of penicillin
    E. uniformly fatal with miliary spread

11. Progressive disseminated histoplasmosis may cause all of the following EXCEPT
    A. spontaneous regression
    B. nasopharyngeal ulcers
    C. hepatomegaly
    D. meningitis
    E. Addison's disease

12. Streptococcal meningitis is usually a complication of
    A. subacute bacterial endocarditis
    B. otitis media
    C. pharyngitis
    D. chorea
    E. cellulitis

13. Deaths due to measles are almost always due to
    A. pneumonia
    B. mastoiditis
    C. meningitis
    D. dehydration
    E. encephalitis

4 / Infectious Diseases, Immunology, and Allergy

14. In pulmonary complications of influenza the most common bacterial invader is
    A. Pneumococcus
    B. *Hemophilus influenzae*
    C. Streptococcus
    D. Staphylococcus
    E. *Neisseria catarrhalis*

15. Food poisoning that results in motor paralysis within 24 hours is most likely due to
    A. *Clostridium botulinum* toxin
    B. staphylococcal toxin
    C. salmonellosis
    D. brucellosis
    E. shigellosis

16. Primary atypical pneumonia is caused by a
    A. bacterium
    B. mycoplasma
    C. fungus
    D. rickettsia
    E. spirochete

17. Complications of infection with *Entamoeba histolytica* include all of the following EXCEPT
    A. liver abscess
    B. renal abscess
    C. meningoencephalitis
    D. intestinal partial obstruction
    E. pleural pulmonary amebiasis

18. Cytomegalovirus infection is best characterized as
    A. always fatal
    B. unresponsive to antibiotics
    C. highly infectious
    D. only acquired
    E. only congenital

19. Herpes zoster is considered to be closely related to
    A. varicella
    B. rubella
    C. rubeola
    D. variola
    E. mumps

20. Brucellosis reservoirs are largely present in
    A. sheep or goats
    B. cats or dogs
    C. parakeets
    D. pigeons
    E. chickens

21. Pustular lesions at the site of the scratch of a cat, followed by malaise, fever, and lymphadenopathy, are likely to be caused by
    A. virus
    B. coccobacilli
    C. acid-fast bacilli
    D. rickettsia
    E. fungus

22. Amebiasis may be complicated by all of the following EXCEPT
    A. liver abscess
    B. pericarditis
    C. chorioretinitis
    D. anemia
    E. neutropenia

23. Allergic rhinitis may be differentiated from infectious rhinitis with the help of all of the following EXCEPT
    A. Wright's stain of the nasal secretions
    B. history of seasonal occurrence
    C. family history
    D. physical examination
    E. age of patient

24. Patients with hay fever
    A. frequently develop asthma
    B. are not improved by moving to different locations
    C. are not more prone to develop upper respiratory infections
    D. are severely disturbed emotionally
    E. can be improved symptomatically only with steroids

25. Humoral antibodies are produced by
    A. B-lymphocytes
    B. T-lymphocytes
    C. macrophages
    D. polymorphonuclear leukocytes
    E. reticuloendothelial cells

26. Chronic vasomotor rhinitis
    A. may result from prolonged exposure to nose drops
    B. is due to allergy to ragweed pollen
    C. is most often due to food allergy
    D. is usually due to only psychosomatic factors
    E. is not associated with eosinophilia in the nasal secretions

27. Laboratory findings in serum sickness may include all of the following EXCEPT
    A. elevated heterophil titer
    B. albuminuria
    C. casts in the urine
    D. rapid sedimentation rate
    E. leukocytosis

28. The most common cause of acute urticaria is
    A. infection
    B. contact allergy
    C. penicillin allergy
    D. food allergy
    E. emotional disturbance

Infectious Diseases, Immunology, and Allergy / 7

29. Delayed hypersensitivity reactions are characterized by
   A. possible transference to another individual by means of serum injections
   B. absence of serum antibody
   C. effect primarily on smooth muscle
   D. presence of high titers of circulating antibody
   E. severe life-threatening reactions

30. In the hereditary form of angioneurotic edema, death is usually
   A. not related to the allergy
   B. an anaphylactic shock reaction
   C. from edema of the glottis
   D. caused by overtreatment
   E. related to stress

31. The most effective treatment for allergic rhinitis is
   A. repeated injection of allergen
   B. antihistamines
   C. steroids
   D. epinephrine
   E. avoidance of allergen

32. Pulmonary cavitation resulting from fungal infection is most likely to be caused by
   A. ringworm
   B. *Cryptococcus neoformans*
   C. *Candida albicans*
   D. mycobacteria
   E. coccidioidomycosis

8 / Infectious Diseases, Immunology, and Allergy

33. Which of the following statements is true regarding tetanus?
   A. Tetanus usually develops within four months following exposure
   B. Tetanus always develops within four hours following exposure in patients who have not been previously immunized
   C. Tetanus may develop many months or years following exposure in susceptible individuals
   D. The usual incubation period for tetanus is 48 hours
   E. Tetanus may be prevented with penicillin

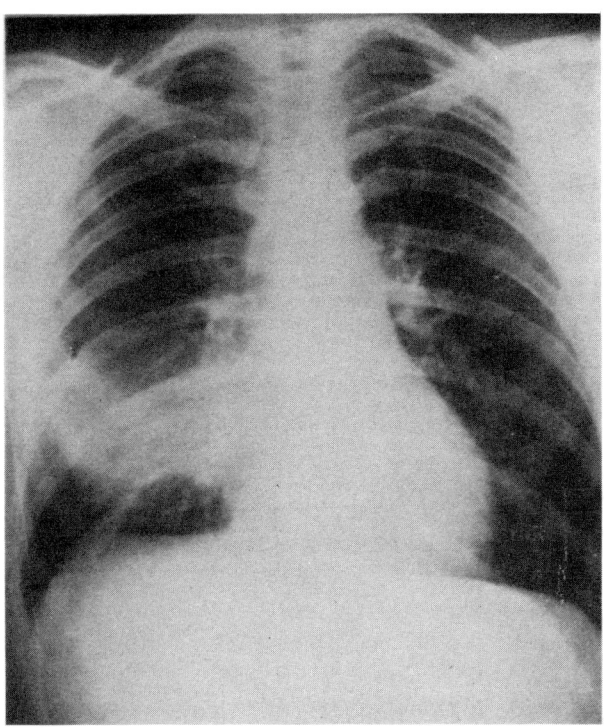

Figure 1.1

Infectious Diseases, Immunology, and Allergy / 9

34. A twenty-five-year-old man is admitted with fever and rust-colored sputum. The chest x-ray is shown in Figure 1.1. What is the most likely diagnosis?
    A. Right middle lobe pneumonia
    B. Loculated pleural effusion
    C. Aspergilloma
    D. Aspiration pneumonia
    E. Right lower lobe pneumonia

35. Most hospital-acquired infections involve
    A. the bloodstream
    B. the lungs
    C. postoperative wounds
    D. the skin
    E. the urinary tract

36. Travellers diarrhea may be markedly reduced by the prophylactic use of
    A. penicillin
    B. doxycycline
    C. chloramphenicol
    D. erythromycin
    E. chloroquine phosphate

37. A renal transplant patient develops severe cough and dyspnea. Bronchial brushings show clusters of cysts that stain with methenamine silver. What is the best treatment?
    A. Amphotericin B
    B. Cephalosporins
    C. Cotrimoxazole
    D. Aminoglycosides
    E. Penicillins

10 / Infectious Diseases, Immunology, and Allergy

DIRECTIONS: Each group of questions below consists of a list of lettered headings followed by a list of numbered words, phrases or statements. For **each** numbered word, phrase or statement, select the **one** lettered heading that is most closely associated with it. Each lettered heading may be selected once, more than once, or not at all.

A. Brucellosis
B. Coccidioidomycosis
C. Histoplasmosis
D. Leprosy
E. Leptospirosis
F. Infectious mononucleosis
G. Tuberculosis
H. Tularemia

38. Oropharyngeal ulcerations

39. Thin-wall pulmonary cavitation

40. Positive Mantoux test

41. Iowa hog farmers

42. Infected rabbits

A. Moniliasis
B. Actinomycosis
C. Sporotrichosis
D. Histoplasmosis
E. Blastomycosis
F. Aspergillosis
G. Cryptococcosis
H. Coccidioidomycosis

43. Tuberculate chlamydospores

44. Thick-walled spherule filled with endospores

45. Sulfur granules

46. Intracellular small oval bodies within polymorphonuclear cells and monocytes on peripheral and bone marrow smears

47. Oval yeastlike cells surrounded by thick capsules outlined clearly in India ink preparations

    A. Toxoplasmosis
    B. Tetanus
    C. Syphilis
    D. Streptococcus
    E. Staphylococcus
    F. Smallpox
    G. Salmonellosis

48. Dark-field examination

49. Congenital brain calcifications

50. Abdominal pain and diarrhea

51. Preventive measures contraindicated in presence of eczema

52. Treated with muscle relaxants

12 / Infectious Diseases, Immunology, and Allergy

DIRECTIONS: Each set of lettered headings below is followed by a list of numbered words or phrases. For each numbered word or phrase select

  A if the item is associated with (A) *only,*
  B if the item is associated with (B) *only,*
  C if the item is associated with *both* (A) *and* (B),
  D if the item is associated with *neither* (A) *nor* (B).

  A. *Mycobacterium tuberculosis*
  B. *Mycobacterium leprae*
  C. Both
  D. Neither

53. Clinically contained by immune reactions for many years

54. Responds to rifampin therapy

55. Acid fast by Ziehl-Neelsen method

56. Therapy may trigger a fatal reaction

DIRECTIONS: For each of the questions or incomplete statements below, **one** or **more** of the answers or completions given is correct. Select

  A if only *1, 2 and 3* are correct,
  B if only *1 and 3* are correct,
  C if only *2 and 4* are correct,
  D if only *4* is correct,
  E if *all* are correct.

57. Aseptic meningitis may be caused by
  1. lymphocytic choriomeningitis
  2. mumps
  3. herpes simplex
  4. tuberculosis

58. Tinea capitis is
   1. caused by fungi
   2. easily diagnosed with a Wood's light
   3. successfully treated with griseofulvin
   4. caused by *Trichophyton* and *Microsporon* species

59. Condylomata lata
   1. are related to venereal warts
   2. occur most frequently on moist areas
   3. are synonymous with condylomata acuminata
   4. occur in secondary syphilis

60. Coxsackie A viruses may cause
   1. paralysis
   2. pneumonitis
   3. common cold
   4. cat-scratch fever

61. Cramps, nausea, vomiting, and fever 48 hours after ingestion of poultry are likely to be due to
   1. *Salmonella typhimurium*
   2. staphylococcus
   3. *Salmonella enteritidis*
   4. botulism

62. In rabies
   1. transmission of the disease is through saliva containing the virus from an infected animal
   2. confirmation of the diagnosis is based on finding Negri bodies in nerve cells
   3. once the first clinical sign of rabies develops, the disease is 100% fatal
   4. bites on the face are more dangerous, because they are closer to the brain

14 / Infectious Diseases, Immunology, and Allergy

Directions Summarized				
A	B	C	D	E
1,2,3 only	1,3 only	2,4 only	4 only	All are correct

63. Toxins
    1. are protein substances elaborated by certain bacteria
    2. are responsible for the pathogenesis of diphtheria, botulism, tetanus, and for the rash in scarlet fever
    3. are neutralized by antitoxins in immune serum, which usually have no effect on the organism producing the toxin
    4. produced in tetanus and botulism are neurotoxic

64. Antibodies to Epstein-Barr virus are found in association with
    1. infectious mononucleosis
    2. nasopharyngeal carcinoma
    3. Burkitt's lymphoma
    4. Hodgkin's disease

65. Complications of disseminated coccidioidomycosis include
    1. erythema nodosum
    2. pleural effusion
    3. phlyctenular conjunctivitis
    4. meningitis

66. Autoantibodies to basement membranes have been well demonstrated to play a role in the pathogenesis of
    1. thyroiditis
    2. myasthenia gravis
    3. hemolytic anemia
    4. Goodpasture's syndrome

67. Hereditary angioneurotic edema is associated with a lack of
    1. serum histamine
    2. basophil migration
    3. complement (C3)
    4. complement (C1 esterase) inhibitor

68. Antigen-antibody complex disease may play a part in the pathogenesis of renal disease in
    1. systemic lupus erythematosus
    2. bacterial endocarditis
    3. chronic glomerulonephritis
    4. mixed cryoglobulin syndromes

69. Injection of horse serum into a sensitized individual may cause
    1. fever
    2. arthralgia
    3. skin eruption
    4. edema

70. Proper therapy for a systemic reaction following the subcutaneous injection of an allergen should include
    1. discontinuation of subsequent injections for three weeks
    2. application of a tourniquet proximal to the injection site
    3. administration of steroids prior to the next injection
    4. administration of epinephrine (1:1000) subcutaneously

71. Significant factors in the pathophysiology of bronchial asthma include
    1. fibrinoid degeneration of the bronchi
    2. swelling of bronchiolar mucosa
    3. microthrombi in the pulmonary capillary bed
    4. narrowing of the lumen by thick sputum

16 / Infectious Diseases, Immunology, and Allergy

Directions Summarized				
A	B	C	D	E
1,2,3 only	1,3 only	2,4 only	4 only	All are correct

72. Allergens commonly responsible for extrinsic asthma are
    1. inhaled organic dusts such as pollens, danders, and spores
    2. house dusts
    3. certain foods such as chocolate and shellfish
    4. certain low molecular weight drugs that may act as haptens

73. Sensitivity to autologous antigen has been demonstrated in
    1. Goodpasture's disease
    2. cold agglutinin syndrome
    3. Hashimoto's disease
    4. degenerative joint disease

74. The symptoms of serum sickness
    1. usually require corticosteroids
    2. are usually self-limited
    3. may be transferred by leukocyte injections
    4. may recur after apparent recovery

75. Laboratory examination in bronchial asthma includes
    1. Curschmann's spirals
    2. Charcot-Leyden crystals
    3. eosinophils in sputum
    4. characteristic chest x-ray

Infectious Diseases, Immunology, and Allergy / 17

76. Which of the following characterizes the syndrome of urticaria and angioedema?
   1. Highest incidence in young adults
   2. Mediated by IgE
   3. Involves mast cell degranulation
   4. Most cases are hereditary

77. Which of the following are characteristic of infection with *Legionella pneumophilia?*
   1. Usually very mild disease
   2. Heavy sputum production
   3. Transmitted by blood transfusion
   4. High fever is common

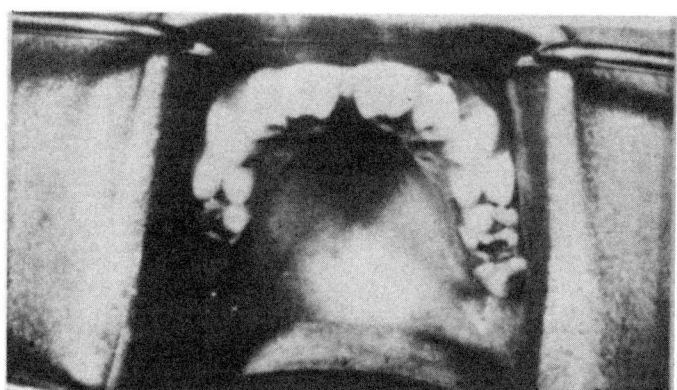

Figure 1.2

78. The dental condition illustrated in Figure 1.2 may be associated with
   1. osteoporosis
   2. depression of the bridge of the nose
   3. Paget's disease of bone
   4. anterior bowing of the tibias

18 / Infectious Diseases, Immunology, and Allergy

DIRECTIONS: This section consists of situations, each followed by a series of questions. Study each situation, and select the **one** best answer to each question following it.

CASE 1 (Questions 79-83): An 18-year-old female visits her physician because of three weeks of malaise, two weeks of fever, and a sore throat. Physical examination shows: pharyngeal infection with enlarged tonsils and a patchy white exudate; enlarged palpable anterior and posterior cervical, axillary, and inguinal lymph nodes; tenderness in the right upper quadrant; and minimal splenomegaly. Laboratory data shows: hemoglobin 14 gm%; hematocrit 42%; platelets 380,000; white blood count 8,500 with 35% segmented neutrophils, 1% eosinophils, and 64% lymphocytes of which 36 were atypical.

79. The most likely diagnosis is
    A. infectious hepatitis
    B. lymphocytic leukemia
    C. infectious mononucleosis
    D. Hodgkin's disease
    E. cat-scratch fever

80. The diagnosis is most likely to be proved by
    A. lymph node biopsy
    B. bone marrow
    C. erythrocyte sedimentation rate
    D. heterophil antibody (sheep cell agglutination) test of Paul-Bunnell
    E. hepatic biopsy

81. The treatment of choice for this disease is
    A. gamma globulin
    B. bed rest
    C. leukeran
    D. chloramphenicol
    E. radiation therapy

Infectious Diseases, Immunology, and Allergy / 19

82. Which one of the following does NOT usually occur as a complication of this disease?
    A. Meningoencephalitis
    B. Guillain-Barré syndrome
    C. Splenic rupture
    D. Jaundice
    E. Hemorrhage

83. Other manifestations of this disease which the patient may develop include all of the following EXCEPT
    A. carditis
    B. maculopapular rash
    C. herpes zoster
    D. jaundice
    E. pinpoint palatal petechiae

CASE 2 (Questions 84-88): A 25-year-old female comes to your office because of malaise for four weeks, fever for two weeks, generalized pain in her joints, and swelling of her vulva. Physical examination reveals a mass in the right inguinal region discharging pus, associated with very marked engorgement of the vulva. Laboratory data shows: hemoglobin 12 gm%; white blood count 12,000 with 55% segmented neutrophils, 45% lymphocytes; total protein 7.4 gm%, with albumin 3.4 gm%, and globulin 4.0 gm%.

84. The most likely diagnosis is
    A. chancroid
    B. syphilis
    C. lymphogranuloma venereum
    D. tuberculous lymphadenitis
    E. granuloma inguinale

85. The most important test in routine diagnosis of the disease is the
    A. culture for acid-fast bacillus
    B. Wassermann test
    C. intradermal Frei test
    D. erythrocyte sedimentation rate
    E. intradermal test with killed Ducrey's bacilli

20 / Infectious Diseases, Immunology, and Allergy

86. A serious complication of this disease is
    A. gumma
    B. rectal stricture
    C. scrofula
    D. sterility
    E. none of these

87. An effective mode of antibiotic therapy is
    A. tetracycline
    B. penicillin
    C. isoniazid
    D. kanamycin
    E. streptomycin

88. All of the following statements concerning this disease are true EXCEPT
    A. the etiologic agent is a virus, which can be cultured on yolk sac cells of the developing chick embryo
    B. some patients have splenomegaly
    C. the first manifestation of the disease is the inguinal bubo, which is very painful
    D. the disease is endemic in the South, particularly among Negroes
    E. a complement fixation test with antigen from virus of chick embryo origin is very sensitive

CASE 3 (Questions 89-93): A 20-year-old woman visits your office because of headache, anorexia, chilly sensations, pain and drawing sensations in both sides of her jaw, and pain in both lower abdominal quadrants. Physical examination reveals: bilateral enlarged parotid glands which are doughy, elastic, and slightly tender; reddened orifice of Stensen's duct; bilateral lower quadrant abdominal tenderness; a temperature of 102°F; and a pulse rate of 92 per minute. Laboratory data shows: Hemoglobin 13 gm%; hematocrit 40%; 9,000 white blood cells, with 35% segmented neutrophils, 7% monocytes, and 58% lymphocytes.

89. The most likely diagnosis is
   A. cervical lymphadenitis
   B. Mikulicz's disease
   C. parotid gland tumor
   D. uveoparotid fever
   E. mumps

90. The patient's abdominal pain and tenderness is most likely due to
   A. mesenteric lymphadenitis
   B. oophoritis
   C. gonorrhea
   D. peritoneal metastases
   E. intestinal hyperperistalsis

91. All of the following are laboratory tests to confirm the diagnosis of epidemic parotitis EXCEPT
   A. complement fixation test during acute and convalescent stage
   B. cutaneous test with suspension of heated inactivated virus
   C. blood culture
   D. hemagglutination inhibition test
   E. serum amylase

92. The best treatment for this disease is
   A. symptomatic
   B. convalescent serum
   C. broad-spectrum antibiotics
   D. sulfonamides
   E. steroids

93. All of the following statements concerning this disease are true EXCEPT
   A. the disease is caused by a filterable virus, is endemic in most large communities, and occurs in epidemics about every seven years
   B. complement-fixing antibody in the circulating blood in adequate titer during convalescence denotes recent infection
   C. the most common complication of this disease in postpubertal boys and men is orchitis
   D. mastitis, pancreatitis, and meningoencephalitis may occur as complications of this disease
   E. in this disease an increased serum amylase is proof of the existence of pancreatitis as a complication

1. Infectious Diseases, Immunology, and Allergy Answers and Comments

1. E. In coccidioidomycosis, probably 1 in 400 infected white males will show dissemination as compared to 1 in 40 Negroes. **(REF. 1, p. 1700)**

2. D. Subacute sclerosing panencephalitis causes involuntary spasmodic movements and progressive mental deterioration, frequently ending in death within a year. **(REF. 1, p. 2102)**

3. E. Enteroviruses include Coxsackie virus group A and B and ECHO viruses, as well as poliomyelitis. **(REF. 1, p. 1663)**

4. C. One-fourth of deaths from influenza are due to pneumonia, with staphylococcus, pneumococcus, and *H. influenzae* the chief organisms. **(REF. 1, p. 1633)**

5. A. Staphylococcal enterotoxin food poisoning is characterized by violent gastrointestinal upset with severe nausea, cramps, vomiting, and diarrhea. **(REF. 1, p. 743)**

6. A. Patients with immune deficiencies or generalized illnesses, pregnant women, infants less than one year old, adults, and all exposed patients should not receive the live rubella vaccine. **(REF. 1, p. 1641)**

7. C. The primary indication of hookworm infection is anemia, which is a combination of blood loss with resulting iron deficiency, and anemia of chronic disease. **(REF. 1, p. 1766)**

8. C. In addition to otitis media, the most common complication of measles, other complications include mastoiditis, pneumonia, bronchitis, encephalitis, and lymphadenitis. **(REF. 1, p. 1636)**

9. E. Granuloma inguinale is not responsive to amphotericin

B. Oral tetracycline, 2 g daily divided into four doses, is the treatment of choice. **(REF. 1, p. 1572)**

10. B. *H. capsulatum* occurs in yeast cell forms and is ingested by the RE system where it produces granulomatous reactions. **(REF. 1, p. 1698)**

11. A. All cases of progressive disseminated histoplasmosis reported to date have been uniformly progressive and fatal. **(REF. 1, p. 1698)**

12. B. Otitis media may result from group A infections of the upper respiratory tract, particularly the mastoid after middle ear disease. **(REF. 1, p. 1445)**

13. A. Pneumonia is an infrequent complication but accounts for over 90% of measles deaths. Giant-cell pneumonia is also seen. **(REF. 1, p. 1636)**

14. D. Staphylococcus is the most common bacterial invader in pulmonary complications of influenza. Pneumonia is the leading cause of death and may also be due to Pneumococcus and *H. influenzae*. **(REF. 1, p. 1633)**

15. A. The incubation period of *C. botulinum* toxin is 12 to 36 hours but ranges from 8 hours to 8 days. There are no sensory symptoms. **(REF. 1, p. 743)**

16. B. Mycoplasmas have no cell walls and have filtration characteristics of viruses but morphologically are closer to bacteria. **(REF. 1, p. 1427)**

17. B. Abscesses develop in the liver, abdominal cavity, spleen, and brain. **(REF. 1, p. 1736)**

18. B. CMV infection is best characterized as unresponsive to antibiotics. In adults it may be asymptomatic and is not a highly communicable disease. **(REF. 1, p. 1649)**

19. A. Immunity to chickenpox follows an attack and appears to protect against a second attack, but zoster seems to be a recrudescence of latent virus. **(REF.** 1, p. 1656)

20. A. Brucellosis is not readily transmitted from man to man but is readily communicable from animals by contact. **(REF.** 1, p. 1535)

21. A. The cause of cat-scratch fever is thought to be a virus closely related to the psittacosis-lymphogranuloma venereum group. **(REF.** 1, p. 1695)

22. E. In addition to liver abscess, pericarditis, chorioretinitis, and anemia, other complications of amebiasis include pleural pulmonary involvement, large granuloma masquerading as neoplasm, or meningoencephalitis. **(REF.** 1, p. 1736)

23. E. Symptoms include pruritus of the eyes, nose and pharynx, but fever, sore throat, and malaise are not seen. **(REF.** 1, p. 1800)

24. A. Sensitivity to a particular allergen such as ragweed may be inherited via an immune response gene. **(REF.** 1, p. 1800)

25. A. B-lymphocytes give rise to plasma cells and antibody-forming cells. **(REF.** 1, p. 1781)

26. A. Chronic vasomotor rhinitis may result from prolonged exposure to nose drops. Vasomotor rhinitis is indistinguishable from allergic rhinitis except for chronicity and absence of geographic and seasonal influence. **(REF.** 1, p. 1802)

27. D. Leukocytosis and circulating plasma cells may be seen, but eosinophilia is uncommon. **(REF.** 1, p. 1815)

28. D. Vasoactive mediators such as histamine, kinins, and SRS-A are released from mast cells, basophils, and other tissues. **(REF.** 1, p. 1796)

29. B. Delayed hypersensitivity is a reaction of T-cells, which have been stimulated by antigen to react against infectious agents, grafts, and tumors. **(REF. 1, p. 1838)**

30. C. In hereditary and angioneurotic edema, the lesions are tense, rounded, nonpitting, and several centimeters in diameter. Edema of the glottis is the usual cause of death. **(REF. 1, p. 1796)**

31. E. Repeated injection with allergen has been in vogue since 1900 and techniques are still controversial. The best treatment for allergic rhinitis is avoidance of allergen. **(REF. 1, p. 1800)**

32. E. Coccidioidomycosis is the usual cause of pulmonary cavitation resulting from fungal infection. A rarefaction may be demonstrable in a pneumonic lesion within ten days of onset. **(REF. 1, p. 1700)**

33. A. In tetanus an acute onset is usual, with pain or tingling at the infection site or reactivity in an apparently healed lesion. **(REF. 1, p. 1499)**

34. A. The x-ray shows a silhouette sign indicating right middle lobe pneumonia. The organism is most likely to be pneumococcus, but care must be taken to consider blockage of the right middle lobe bronchus. **(REF. 1, pp. 1416-1441)**

35. E. Most hospital-acquired infections involve the urinary tract, accounting for about 35% of infections. Postoperative wounds account for 20%, and pulmonary and bloodstream infections account for 15% each. **(REF. 1, pp. 1402-1404)**

36. B. Doxycycline 200 mg on the day of travel followed by 100 mg daily for three weeks markedly reduced the incidence of diarrhea in Peace Corps volunteers in double-blind studies. **(REF. 1, p. 1415)**

37. C. The patient is infected with pneumocystis organisms, invading an immunocompromised host. The treatment of choice is trimethoprim sulfamethoxazole which is equally effective as pentamidine. Cotrimoxazole combines the above two drugs. **(REF.** 1, pp. 1742-1744)

38. C. In histoplasmosis, oropharyngeal ulcerations begin as solitary indurated plaques with no pain present at first, although eventually pain becomes deep-seated. **(REF.** 1, p. 1698)

39. B. In coccidioidomycosis, hemoptysis may call attention to cavitations or patients may complain of pain at the cavity site. **(REF.** 1, p. 1700)

40. G. The intracutaneous tuberculin test with PPD is read for evidence of delayed hypersensitivity at 48 hours. **(REF.** 1, p. 1541)

41. A. Brucellosis is prevalent in midwestern hog-raising states, in Texas, and in California. **(REF.** 1, p. 1535)

42. H. Tularemia can be acquired through direct contact with an infected rabbit which may occur in preparation or cooking inadequately. **(REF.** 1, p. 1524)

43. D. Parasitization of yeast cell forms of *H. capsulatum* causes a granulomatous reaction in the RE system in histoplasmosis. **(REF.** 1, p. 1698)

44. H. The sporangial or spherule form found in animals is poorly adapted to aerial transfer, since coccidioidomycosis is not contagious. **(REF.** 1, p. 1700)

45. B. Actinomycosis is characterized by chronic inflammatory induration, sinus formation, and sulfur granules. **(REF.** 1, p. 1532)

46. D. In histoplasmosis the yeast cells multiply by budding and are 3 to 4 microns in diameter. **(REF.** 1, p. 1698)

47. G. Cryptococcosis is a pulmonary infection with encapsulated yeast with a special predilection for the central nervous system. **(REF.** 1, p. 1703)

48. C. On dark-field examination, *Treponema pallidum* (the spirochete which causes syphilis) is a thin, delicate organism with tapering ends and 6 to 14 spirals. **(REF. 1, p. 1573)**

49. A. Congenital toxoplasmosis is initiated in utero usually as a complication of a primary infection. **(REF. 1, p. 1739)**

50. G. Salmonellosis is an acute infection resulting from ingestion of food containing bacteria and is characterized by abdominal pain and diarrhea. **(REF. 1, p. 1507)**

51. F. Preventive measures are contraindicated in the presence of eczema in smallpox. They are also contraindicated in leukemia, lymphoma, dysgammaglobulinemias, and immunosuppressed patients. **(REF. 1, p. 1658)**

52. B. Patients with tetanus develop hypertonus, seizures, respiratory distress, and asphyxia unless they are treated with muscle relaxants. **(REF. 1, p. 1499)**

53. C. Tuberculoid leprosy generally presents as a single large plaque that is very well defined. Primary infection tuberculosis is usually confined to the lung and lymph nodes. **(REF. 1, pp. 1542, 1559)**

54. C. Rifampin has a high order of effectiveness in TB and is a first-line drug in many countries. As primary and secondary resistance to dapsone is described in leprosy, rifampin is becoming a drug of choice for the first 18 months, combined with dapsone. **(REF. 1, pp. 1545, 1560)**

55. C. *M. tuberculosis* and *M. leprae* are both acid-alcohol fast by the ZN technique. *M. leprae* has not yet been successfully cultured in vitro, but can be grown in the footpads of mice. **(REF. 1, pp. 1539, 1557)**

56. B. Effective antileprosy therapy may trigger a reactional state known as erythema nodosum leprosum in patients with high bacterial loads. Serious morbidity or death may result. **(REF. 1, p. 1559)**

Infectious Diseases, Immunology, and Allergy / 29

57. A. Aseptic meningitis is a syndrome characterized by inflammation and lymphocytic infiltration of the meninges. It is not caused by tuberculosis. **(REF. 1, p. 1647)**

58. E. Tinea capitus is characterized by partial alopecia, loss of luster of the hair, and inflammation of the scalp. All four statements listed are correct. **(REF. 1, p. 2268)**

59. C. Condylomata lata are raised, table-topped or mushroom-like papules occurring most frequently on moist areas about the genitalia or rectum in patients with secondary syphilis. **(REF. 1., p. 1577)**

60. A. In addition to paralysis, pneumonitis, and the common cold, Coxsackie A viruses also may cause summer febrile illness, aseptic meningitis, herpangina, and exanthem. **(REF. 1, p. 1663)**

61. B. Poultry, meats, eggs, and egg products have a high prevalence of contamination of *S. typhimurium* and *S. enteritides*. **(REF. 1, p. 1507)**

62. E. All four statements about rabies are correct. Rabies is transmitted by the bite of an infected animal and causes hyperexcitability or apathy, paralysis, and death. **(REF. 1, pp. 2097–2100)**

63. E. All four statements are true about toxins. Their effect usually requires a very small amount of toxin, so that one millionth of a milliliter can cause neurologic effects in botulism. **(REF. 1, p. 1498)**

64. A. The association of antibodies to EBV with infectious mononucleosis, nasopharyngeal carcinoma, and Burkitt's lymphoma is strong, but etiology has not yet been established. **(REF. 1, pp. 953, 1651)**

65. E. Pulmonary cavitation may develop into a large, thin-walled cavity and is a more worrisome complication of coccidioidomycosis than those listed. **(REF. 1, p. 1700)**

66. D. Other examples where these antibodies play a pathogenetic role are Hashimoto's disease, autoimmune hemolytic anemia, and thrombocytopenias. **(REF. 1, p. 381)**

67. D. Complement (C1 esterase) inhibitor deficiency favors formation of C2a and C3a and, indirectly, plasmin and kallikrein. **(REF. 1, p. 14)**

68. E. All factors listed are true of antigen-antibody complex disease. Mixed cryoglobulins are made up of IgG and IgM complexed as antigen and antibody. **(REF. 1, p. 1779)**

69. E. Injection of horse serum into a sensitized person may cause all four conditions listed. Serum sickness represents a hypersensitivity reaction to foreign protein or to drugs. **(REF. 1, p. 1815)**

70. C. These systemic reactions are uncommon and easily managed in the office if detected, but if the patient leaves too soon it could be dangerous. Proper therapy includes application of a tourniquet proximal to the injection site and administration of epinephrine subcutaneously. **(REF. 1, p. 1816)**

71. C. Narrowing of the lumen by thick sputum and swelling of bronchiolar mucosa are significant factors in bronchial asthma. There is a constant state of hyperreactivity of the bronchi, during which exposure to an irritant precipitates an asthmatic attack. **(REF. 1, p. 365)**

72. E. Allergic factors, including all those listed, are presumed to be active in most cases of asthma, either to induce hyperreactivity or to trigger attacks. **(REF. 1, p. 365)**

73. A. Sensitivity to autologous antigen has not been demonstrated in degenerative joint disease. In Goodpasture's disease, antibodies are reative with the basement membrane of lung and kidney. **(REF. 1, p. 381)**

74. C. The symptoms of serum sickness are usually self-limited and may recur after apparent recovery. The natural course is one to three weeks, so that steroid toxicity does not occur before treatment is stopped. (**REF.** 1, p. 1815)

75. A. Laboratory examination in bronchial asthma does not include characteristic chest x-ray; chest x-ray shows hyperinflation. Peripheral blood often shows eosinophilia and slight granulocytosis. (**REF.** 1, p. 365)

76. A. Urticaria and angioedema involve the skin, respiratory tract, and gastrointestinal and possibly cardiovascular systems. It is most common in young adults and is attributed to an immediate-type immunologic reaction. Most cases are idiopathic. (**REF.** 1, pp. 1796-1799)

77. D. Legionnaire's disease is transmitted by airborne routes and causes a severe disease characterized by dry cough and fevers. There is a 15% to 20% mortality rate. (**REF.** 8, pp. 1091, 1225)

78. C. The figure illustrates Hutchinson's teeth which is a manifestation of late congenital syphilis. This may be associated with cardiovascular and neurologic manifestations as well as "saddle nose" and "sabre shins." (**REF.** 1, p. 1579)

79. C. Infectious mononucleosis is an acute, self-limited infection of the lymphatic system, probably by the EB virus. (**REF.** 1, p. 1651)

80. D. The presence of EB virus antibody at a 1:10 dilution by the indirect immunofluorescence test indicates immunity. (**REF.** 1, p. 1652)

81. B. Antibiotics are of no avail, except that penicillin may eradicate streptococcal carriage if present. Bed rest is the treatment of choice. (**REF.** 1, p. 1653)

82. E. Hemorrhage is not a usual complication of infectious mononucleosis. Over 90% of cases are benign and uncomplicated, but liver involvement is clinical in 5% to 10%. (**REF.** 1, p. 1652)

83. C. Herpes zoster is not a manifestation of infectious mononucleosis. Neurologic manifestations include meningitis and encephalitis in one to two percent of cases. (**REF.** 1, p. 1652)

84. C. Lymphogranuloma venereum is a viral disease usually acquired through sexual contact, with an evanescent initial lesion and lymphadenopathy. (**REF.** 1, pp. 1571–1572)

85. C. The intradermal Frei test is the most important test in routine diagnosis of lymphogranuloma venereum. The antigen is made from infected yolk and chick embryo; 0.1 ml of antigen is injected intradermally. (**REF.** 1, p. 1571)

86. B. Rectal stricture is commonly found without a history or other clinical findings of the disease, most often in females. (**REF.** 1, p. 1572)

87. A. Best results are obtained from tetracycline therapy in early acute cases, but little benefit is obtained after scarring begins. (**REF.** 1, p. 1572)

88. C. The bubo usually appears in 10 to 30 days, although several months may elapse. (**REF.** 1, p. 1571)

89. E. Mumps is an acute communicable infection with localized swelling of one or more salivary glands. (**REF.** 1, pp. 1642–1644)

90. B. Pain referring to either or both lower quadrants is common when oophoritis is present. (**REF.** 1, p. 1643)

91. C. Complement fixation tests are run on specimens drawn as soon after onset as possible and then at the end of the third week. (**REF.** 1, p. 1641)

92. A. Antibiotics, sulfas, steroids, and mumps convalescent sera are of no value. (**REF.** 1, p. 1643)

93. E. Serum amylase is elevated in 96% of cases because of parotitis, not pancreatitis. (**REF.** 1, p. 1642)

2. Diseases of the Digestive System

DIRECTIONS: Each of the questions or incomplete statements below is followed by five suggested answers or completions. Select the **one** that is **best** in each case.

94. All of the following are characteristic of hepatitis B antigen EXCEPT that it is
    A. detected in the early acute phase
    B. found in epidemiologically documented short-incubation hepatitis
    C. prevalent in some tropical countries
    D. seen in Down's syndrome
    E. localized in liver cell nuclei

95. Characteristically, carcinoid tumors
    A. are more common in women
    B. produce hypertension
    C. produce jaundice
    D. produce steatorrhea
    E. are multiple in 15% to 25% of cases

96. Argentaffin tumors of the small intestine
    A. are only found in the appendix
    B. produce pheochromocytomas
    C. produce carcinoid syndrome
    D. do not metastisize
    E. are always single

34 / Diseases of the Digestive System

97. Characteristically, cancer of the esophagus
    A. usually occurs in the upper third
    B. is more common in females
    C. has a five-year cure rate of 20%
    D. may be either adenocarcinoma or squamous cell carcinoma
    E. always presents with early dysphagia

98. The most reliable method of measuring steatorrhea is
    A. xylose absorption
    B. Schilling test
    C. x-ray studies
    D. stool fat quantitation
    E. small intestinal biopsy

99. Which of the following is a feature of Meckel's diverticulum?
    A. It is more common in females
    B. It is located in the colon
    C. It rarely ulcerates
    D. It arises from Gartner's duct
    E. None of the above

100. A characteristic of Plummer-Vinson syndrome is
    A. increased frequency in men
    B. esophageal diverticula
    C. hypochromic anemia
    D. spontaneous esophageal rupture
    E. none of the above

101. Acquired lactase deficiency is seen in association with all of the following EXCEPT
    A. nontropical sprue
    B. tropical sprue
    C. regional enteritis
    D. ulcerative colitis
    E. viral gastroenteritis

102. Clinical characteristics of Whipple's disease include all of the following EXCEPT
    A. women are usually affected
    B. arthritis
    C. diarrhea
    D. progressive wasting
    E. skin pigmentation

103. Nontropical sprue includes all of the following features EXCEPT
    A. decrease in intestinal disaccharidases
    B. weight loss
    C. mononuclear infiltrate in mucosa
    D. increase in pancreatic enzymes
    E. response to gluten-free diet

104. The most sensitive technique for early diagnosis of gastric cancer is
    A. barium swallow and UGI series
    B. fiberoptic endoscopy
    C. clinical history
    D. sputum cytology
    E. physical examination

105. Which of the following conditions is associated with impaired hepatic uptake of bilirubin?
    A. Crigler-Najjar syndrome
    B. Dubin-Johnson syndrome
    C. Rotor's syndrome
    D. Gilbert's syndrome
    E. Pregnanediol therapy

106. Dark-brown spots in the lips and palate associated with Peutz-Jeghers syndrome may indicate
    A. intestinal polyposis
    B. Addison's disease
    C. lead poisoning
    D. malignant melanoma
    E. gastric ulcers

36 / Diseases of the Digestive System

107. Glucuronyl transferase is an enzyme important in
    A. uptake of bilirubin in the liver cell
    B. conjugation of bilirubin
    C. breakdown of hemoglobin
    D. formation of delta-amino levulinic acid
    E. excretion of bilirubin

108. Postprandial postgastrectomy syndromes may be associated with all of the following EXCEPT
    A. symptoms 20 minutes after eating
    B. palpitation and sweating
    C. functional hypoglycemia
    D. relief with frequent small meals
    E. prolonged vomiting

109. The occurrence of acute diarrhea in several patients within 24 hours of eating the same meal is evidence of
    A. ingestion of a preformed toxin
    B. ingestion of amebae
    C. infectious colitis
    D. arsenic poisoning
    E. viral gastroenteritis

110. Characteristics of hepatoma include all of the following EXCEPT
    A. commonly metastasize
    B. poor prognosis
    C. predisposing cirrhosis
    D. markedly elevated alkaline phosphatase
    E. more common in males

111. Ascitic fluid in cirrhosis of the liver would be expected to show
    A. hemorrhage
    B. protein greater than 2.5 gm per 100 ml
    C. positive malignant cytology
    D. specific gravity less than 1.016
    E. more than 1000 white cells per cubic mm

Diseases of the Digestive System / 37

112. Which of the following is true of common duct stones?
    A. All originate in the gallbladder
    B. They always produce jaundice
    C. Jaundice is always constant
    D. Jaundice can be painless
    E. None of the above

113. Patients with anorexia nervosa may manifest all of the following EXCEPT
    A. extreme emaciation
    B. loss of pubic/axillary hair
    C. decreased blood pressure
    D. signs of vitamin deficiency
    E. psychiatric disturbance

114. Diarrhea and cramping with postprandial vasomotor phenomena with concomitant cardiovascular findings should suggest
    A. abdominal angina
    B. pheochromocytoma
    C. carcinoid syndrome
    D. hyperlipemia
    E. congestive heart failure and small bowel ulceration

115. The diagnosis of achalasia (cardiospasm) includes all of the following EXCEPT
    A. symptoms of dysphagia
    B. symptoms of regurgitation
    C. hyposensitive Mecholyl test
    D. smooth narrowing of lower esophagus
    E. lack of resistance to passage of esophagoscope through the narrowed segment

116. Which one of the following cations is present in gastric juice in a larger concentration than in blood plasma?
    A. Sodium
    B. Potassium
    C. Magnesium
    D. Calcium
    E. Lithium

38 / Diseases of the Digestive System

117. Mechanical narrowing of the esophageal lumen causing dysphagia is commonly caused by any of the following EXCEPT
    A. squamous cell carcinoma of the esophagus
    B. adenocarcinoma of the cardia of the stomach
    C. reflux esophagitis
    D. lye ingestion
    E. motor system disease

118. Zollinger-Ellison syndrome is associated with all of the following EXCEPT
    A. 12-hour nocturnal secretion of gastric juice over 2 liters
    B. diffusion of 50% of tumors throughout the pancreas
    C. malignancy of 50% of tumors
    D. recurrent peptic ulcerations
    E. small incidence of hypoglycemia

119. When a woman with active ulcerative colitis becomes pregnant the colitis will probably
    A. not be affected
    B. become quiescent
    C. become worse
    D. become worse in the third trimester
    E. cause a high fetal mortality

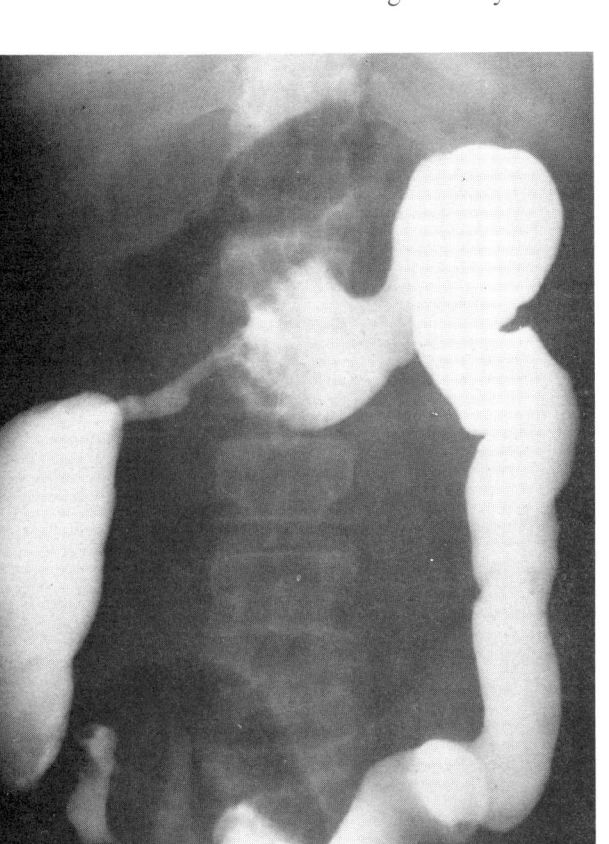

Figure 2.1

120. A 35-year-old Caucasian male presents with a long history of fulminant diarrhea and rectal bleeding (Fig. 2.1). What is your diagnosis?
   A. Toxic megacolon
   B. Amebic colitis
   C. Appendicitis
   D. Ischemic colitis
   E. Annular carcinoma

40 / Diseases of the Digestive System

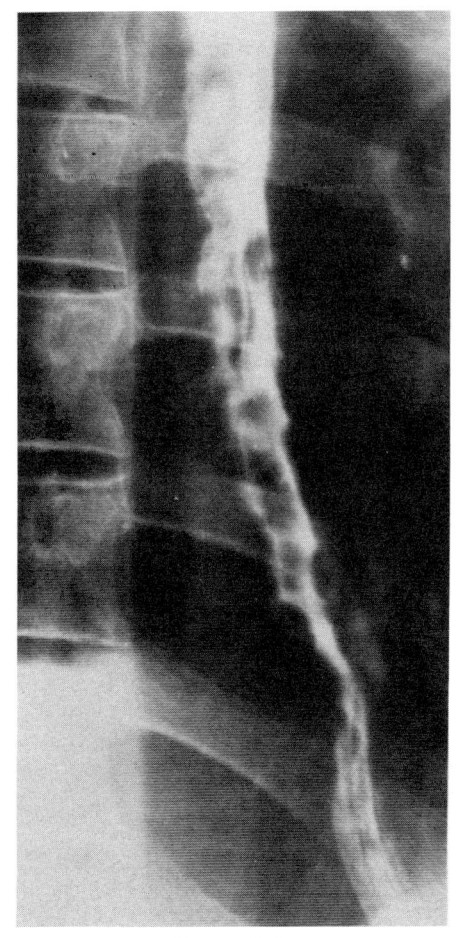

Figure 2.2

121. A 45-year-old Irishman with a long history of alcoholic intake comes into the emergency room with upper gastrointestinal bleeding (Fig. 2.2). What is your diagnosis?
    A. Esophageal varices
    B. Esophageal carcinoma
    C. Foreign body
    D. Tertiary waves
    E. Barrett's esophagus

Diseases of the Digestive System / 41

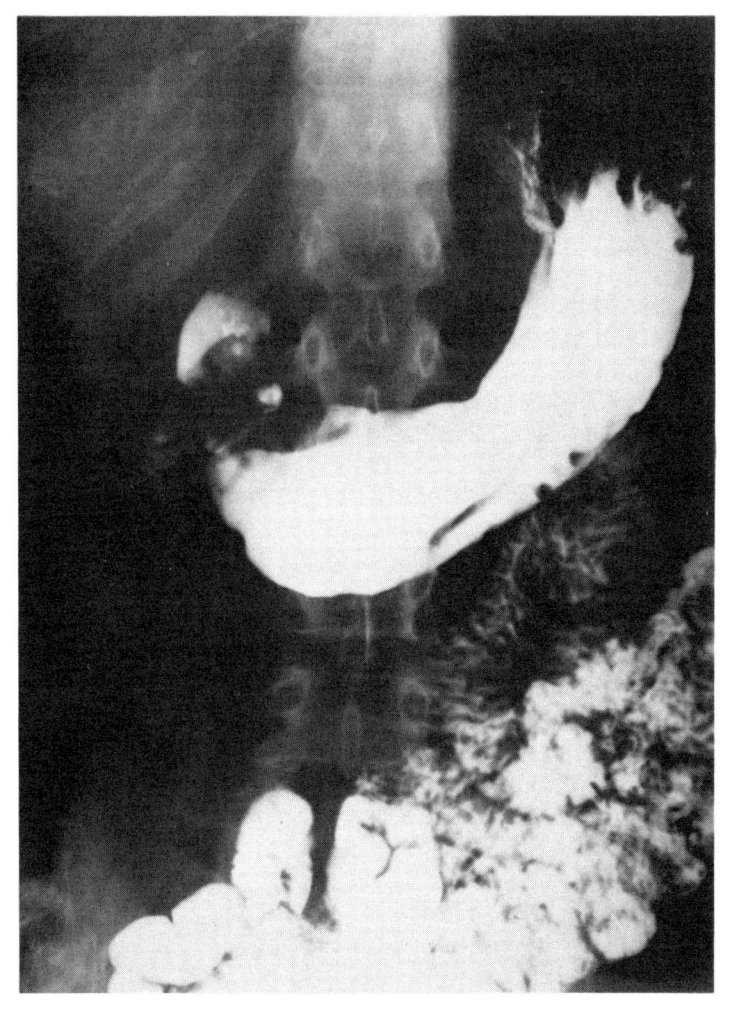

Figure 2.3

122. A 40-year-old taxicab driver presents with worsening epigastric pain (Fig. 2.3). What is your diagnosis?
 A. Benign gastric ulcer
 B. Malignant gastric ulcer
 C. Duodenal ulcer
 D. Normal
 E. Hiatus hernia

A. Hepatitis A
B. Hepatitis B
C. Non-A, Non-B hepatitis
D. Chronic persistent hepatitis
E. Chronic active hepatitis

123. Associated with alpha-1-antitrypsin deficiency

124. Causative agent appears to be a 27 nm RNA particle

125. The major cause of post-transfusion hepatitis

126. Commonly transmitted amongst the sexually promiscuous, especially male homosexuals

127. A nonprogressive inflammatory process largely confined to the portal areas with no significant stromal collapse

A. Ulcerative colitis
B. Crohn's colitis
C. Amebic colitis
D. Pseudomembranous colitis
E. Irritable bowel syndrome

128. *Clostridium difficile* infection is a frequent concomitant

129. An important public health problem among homosexual men

130. The most common gastrointestinal disorder in Western societies

131. Proctocolectomy and ileostomy are indicated with failure of medical therapy

132. A tender mass in the right lower quadrant may simulate appendicitis

---

DIRECTIONS: Each set of lettered headings below is followed by a list of numbered words or phrases. For each numbered word or phrase select
    A if the item is associated with (A) *only,*
    B if the item is associated with (B) *only,*
    C if the item is associated with *both* (A) *and* (B),
    D if the item is associated with *neither* (A) *nor* (B).

    A. Benign gastric ulcer
    B. Malignant gastric ulcer
    C. Both
    D. Neither

133. Associated with bezoars

134. Carman's (meniscus) sign

135. Extension of the tumor beyond the contour of the curvature

136. Prepyloric ulcer

137. Frequently complete healing in four to six weeks

44 / Diseases of the Digestive System

    A. Regional ileitis
    B. Ulcerative colitis
    C. Both
    D. Neither

138. Fistulas occur as complications

139. Granulomas of the submucosa

140. Increased incidence of carcinoma

141. Frequently arthritis occurs

142. "Skip areas" on x-ray

DIRECTIONS: For each of the questions or incomplete statements below, **one** or **more** of the answers or completions given is correct. Select
    A if only *1, 2 and 3* are correct,
    B if only *1 and 3* are correct,
    C if only *2 and 4* are correct,
    D if only *4* is correct,
    E if *all* are correct.

---

143. Acute pancreatitis tends to occur in patients with
    1. alcoholism
    2. peptic ulcer
    3. dietary debauchery
    4. lysinuria

144. The physical signs of pancreatic pseudocyst include
    1. increased bowel sounds
    2. jaundice
    3. right upper abdominal mass
    4. atelectasis of the left lung base

Diseases of the Digestive System / 45

145. The actions of pure gastrin include
    1. stimulation of pepsin secretion
    2. stimulation of gastric motility
    3. increased volume output by the pancreas
    4. increased flow of hepatic bile

146. The gastric phase of gastric secretion encompasses
    1. activation of local cholinergic reflexes
    2. a direct effect of secretin
    3. secretion of antral gastrin
    4. increased vagal tone over long vagal tracts

147. Cholestatic jaundice is associated with
    1. predominantly conjugated hyperbilirubinemia
    2. minimal biochemical changes of parenchymal liver damage
    3. a moderate to marked increase in the serum alkaline phosphatase
    4. a moderate to marked increase in SGOT

148. Evidence of marked obstruction due to peptic ulcer might include
    1. 50 cc of gastric juice retention
    2. metabolic acidosis
    3. urine of a low specific gravity
    4. an elevated hematocrit

149. Disorders associated with protein-losing enteropathy include
    1. gastric carcinoma
    2. nontropical sprue
    3. ulcerative colitis
    4. congestive heart failure

150. The colon and rectum are supplied by
    1. sympathetic nerves
    2. parasympathetic nerves
    3. sensory fibers
    4. motor fibers

46 / Diseases of the Digestive System

Directions Summarized				
A	B	C	D	E
1,2,3 only	1,3 only	2,4 only	4 only	All are correct

151. Bile salts
1. form micelles
2. shift the pH optimum of lipases
3. help fat absorption
4. bind sugars

152. Characteristics of acute necrotizng (membranous) enterocolitis often include
1. previous antibiotic therapy
2. associated insult to circulation
3. high fatality rate
4. streptococcal invasion

153. Vomiting of black or "coffee-grounds" vomitus usually indicates
1. vomiting immediately after bleeding
2. vomiting several hours after bleeding
3. bleeding distal to the jejunum
4. bleeding proximal to the jejunum

154. Features of biliary cirrhosis include
1. malignant clinical course
2. marked hepatomegaly
3. nonobstructive-type jaundice
4. elevated serum lipids

155. The small bowel mucosal biopsy is normal in
1. postgastrectomy steatorrhea
2. tropical sprue
3. pancreatic steatorrhea
4. Whipple's disease

156. The string sign in ileitis is seen
  1. in the stenotic phase of the disease
  2. in the nonstenotic phase of the disease
  3. to distend slightly
  4. to be completely rigid and nondistensible

157. Volvulus of the intestines occurs most frequently at which of the following sites?
  1. Ileum
  2. Cecum
  3. Sigmoid flexure
  4. Stomach

48 / Diseases of the Digestive System

2. Diseases of the Digestive System Answers and Comments

94. B Hepatitis B antigen is not found in epidemiologically documented short-incubation hepatitis. Three types of antigen particles have been identified in serum. Heating of serum destroys infectivity but not antigenicity. **(REF. 1, p. 780)**

95. E. Carcinoid tumors are multiple in 15% to 25% of cases. Primary carcinoid tumors of the appendix are common but rarely metastasize. Those in the large colon may metastasize but do not function. **(REF. 1, p. 1312)**

96. C. Argentaffin tumors are the most common epithelial tumors of the small bowel, are often multiple, and cause carcinoid syndrome when the liver is invaded. **(REF. 1, p. 1312)**

97. D. Lesions in the upper two-thirds of the esophagus are squamous, but in the distal esophagus over half are adenocarcinomas. **(REF. 1, p. 1048)**

98. D. Greater than 6 gm of stool fat per 24 hours indicates malabsorption or maldigestion. **(REF. 1, p. 682)**

99. E. Only a small percentage of Meckel's diverticula cause trouble, but they must be thought of in every case of GI hemorrhage and obstruction. **(REF. 1, p. 667)**

100. C. Iron is usually effective in treating hypochromic anemia. Instrumentation of the esophagus is rarely required. **(REF. 1, p. 849)**

101. E. Viral gastroenteritis is not seen in association with acquired lactase deficiency. Lactase deficiency occurs in a wide variety of GI diseases in which there is evidence of mucosal disease. **(REF. 1, p. 693)**

102. A. Whipple's disease is unusual in women and occurs predominantly in men of middle age. **(REF. 1, p. 696)**

103. D. Severe mucosal damage leads to decrease in secretin and cholecystokinin and decreased pancreatic secretion. **(REF. 1, p. 694)**

104. B. On fiberoptic endoscopy, cancers of less than 1 cm can be visualized in 60% of cases, and accuracy is over 90% for all gastric cancers. **(REF. 1, p. 655)**

105. D. Gilbert's syndrome is associated with impaired hepatic uptake of bilirubin. Uptake of bilirubin by the liver cell involves dissociation of the pigment from albumin and binding to cytoplasmic proteins (Y and Z). **(REF. 1, p. 773)**

106. A. Intestinal polyposis is a possible indication of Peutz-Jeghers syndrome associated with dark-brown spots on the lips and palate. There is characteristic distribution of pigment around lips, nose, eyes, and hands. **(REF. 1, p. 1050)**

107. B. Conjugation of bilirubin occurs in the endoplasmic reticulum of the hepatocytes. **(REF. 1, p. 772)**

108. E. Prolonged vomiting is not associated with postprandial postgastrectomy syndromes. The early syndrome may be due to fluid loss into the intestine, release of serotonin or kinins, or enteric glucagon release. **(REF. 1, p. 663)**

109. A. Diarrhea in several patients after 24 to 48 hours of eating the same meal indicates ingestion of a salmonella. **(REF. 1, p. 1507)**

110. A. Hepatomas usually do not metastasize. In parts of Africa and Asia hepatomas comprise 20% to 30% of all malignant conditions. **(REF. 1, p. 812)**

111. D. Ascitic fluid in cirrhosis of the liver shows a specific gravity less than 1.016. Protein is less than 2.5%, and the gross appearance is straw colored. **(REF. 1, p. 806)**

112. D. Jaundice can be painless, or it may give rise to severe pain, chills, and fever. **(REF. 1, p. 764)**

113. B. Anorexia nervosa occurs 20 times more often in females than males. It does not cause loss of pubic/axillary hair. **(REF. 1, p. 1379)**

114. C. These signs suggest carcinoid syndrome. Flushing, lacrimation, tachycardia, and telangicctasia may also be associated. **(REF. 1, p. 1312)**

115. C. Severe achalasia may have minimal dysphagia, delayed regurgitation, persistent substernal pain, and cachexia. A hyposensitive Mecholyl test is not diagnostic of achalasia. **(REF. 1, p. 627)**

116. B. Potassium is present in gastric juice in a larger concentration than in blood plasma. Concentrations of potassium remain within a narrow range. **(REF. 1, p. 661)**

117. E. Squamous cell carcinoma accounts for 95% of true esophageal tumors, but often adenocarcinoma of the stomach causes esophageal symptoms. Motor system disease is not a cause of mechanical narrowing of the esophageal lumen. **(REF. 1, p. 1048)**

118. B. Diffusion of 50% of tumors throughout the pancreas is not a feature of the Zollinger-Ellison syndrome. In 20% of cases, multiple endocrine adenomas are present in parathyroid, pituitary adrenal, or thyroid. **(REF. 1, p. 641)**

119. C. A woman with active ulcerative colitis who becomes pregnant usually becomes worse; however, about 70% of patients have remissions with medical treatment. **(REF. 1, p. 711)**

120. E. The carcinoma has occurred in a patient with ulcerative colitis. The barium enema shows a long, constricting lesion in the transverse colon with the whole colon devoid of haustral markings. Some pressure effects are seen in the ileum due to metastases. The diagnosis of ulcerative colitis is made from the clinical symptoms and proctosigmoidoscopic examination of an abnormally inflamed colonic mucosa. **(REF. 1, p. 727)**

Diseases of the Digestive System / 51

121. A. In esophageal varices the esophageal folds are thick and tortuous, giving rise to a wormy or worm-eaten appearance. The radiographic picture would vary with the severity of the varices, as well as the distention of the esophagus. When varices are severe, they should be appreciated in any projection. The left anterior oblique projection is most ideal for its demonstration. **(REF.** 1, p. 805)

122. A. In benign gastric ulcer an ulcer niche is present in the prepyloric area, with folds radiating to and extending up to the margin of the niche with a halo around it. The differentiation between benignity and malignancy may be difficult at times, but proper use of radiographic criteria could boost the accuracy to 98%. In the presence of an ulcer niche a Hampton line, which is an ulcer collar, or a mound should be sought on a profile view. **(REF.** 1, p. 643)

123. E. Chronic active hepatitis requires a biopsy for diagnosis as it is essential to establish a specific cause if possible, such as alpha-1-antitrypsin deficiency, Wilson's disease, or ethanol. **(REF.** 1, pp. 790–792)

124. A. The causative agent of hepatitis A virus is a 27 nm diameter RNA virus which, although similar to other picornaviruses, is not cytopathogenic in tissue culture. Hepatitis B is associated with the 42 nm DNA particle. **(REF.** 1, p. 779)

125. C. Non-A, non-B hepatitis is the major cause of post-transfusion hepatitis. It occurs in approximately 5 to 10 cases per 1000 transfusions and is especially transmitted in clotting factor concentrates. **(REF.** 1, p. 783)

126. B. The hepatitis B virus is present in virtually all body fluids and excreta and is therefore transmitted by sexual contact, as well as by transfusion or exposure of health care workers. **(REF.** 1, p. 782)

127. D. There is little or no periportal or lobular hepatitis, and fibrosis and cirrhosis are absent. This condition may be entirely asymptomatic or associated with nonspecific symptoms. **(REF.** 1, p. 789)

52 / Diseases of the Digestive System

128. D. Pseudomembranous colitis usually follows recent antibiotic exposure. *C. difficile* is found as normal flora in some patients. The mechanism is toxin-mediated without invasion of the intestinal wall. **(REF. 1, p. 1497)**

129. C. Spread may be by the fecal-oral route. *Entamoeba histolytica* may invade the bowel wall to produce colitis and spread to distant sites such as the liver. **(REF. 1, p. 1737)**

130. E. This condition consists of abdominal discomfort, alterations of bowel habit, but no demonstrable organic cause. Up to 50% of all referrals for consultation in gastroenterology are for irritable bowel syndrome. **(REF. 1, p. 669)**

131. A. Indications for total colectomy in ulcerative colitis include perforation, colonic carcinoma, and massive hemorrhage. **(REF. 1, p. 710)**

132. B. Surgical exploration is commonly employed to distinguish the two conditions. Symptoms in favor of Crohn's disease include diarrhea, weight loss, and a history of aphthous ulcerations of the mouth. **(REF. 1, p. 714)**

133. D. The vast majority of gastric ulcers are benign; about 7% with no clear diagnosis will prove malignant. Neither benign nor malignant gastric ulcers are associated with bezoars. **(REF. 1, p. 643)**

134. B. X-ray examination and fiberoptic endoscopy are the two most valuable investigations of malignant gastric ulcer. **(REF. 1, p. 643)**

135. C. The defect extends beyond the projected wall of the stomach in both, but it is smooth and oval when benign. **(REF. 1, p. 643)**

136. C. Both benign and malignant gastric ulcers are most often antral and are usually single and on the lesser curvative. **(REF. 1, p. 643)**

137. A. Benign ulcers should reduce by 50% in two to three weeks at repeat examination, and they often heal completely in four to six weeks. **(REF. 1, p. 643)**

138. C. Fistulas occur in both but favor the diagnosis of granulomatous disease. **(REF. 1, pp. 703, 711)**

139. A. Endothelial cell proliferation in lymphatics, giant cell aggregation in submucosa, and arteriolar changes are seen in regional ileitis. **(REF. 1, pp. 703, 711)**

140. B. Factors increasing the risk of carcinoma in ulcerative colitis are disease duration, pancolitis, and family history. **(REF. 1, pp. 703, 711)**

141. C. Acute arthritis may occur in both, involving large joints and without a rheumatoid factor. **(REF. 1 pp. 703, 711)**

142. A. In addition to "skip areas" on x-ray, stiffening of submucosae, separation of tubular loops, and narrowing of the lumen with dilatation of the proximal bowel are other signs of regional ileitis. **(REF. pp. 703, 711)**

143. E. Acute pancreatitis most commonly follows alcoholism or biliary tract disease and tends to occur in patients with peptic ulcer, dietary debauchery, and lysinuria. It may be due to mumps or viral hepatitis. **(REF. 1, p. 733)**

144. C. Jaundice and atelectasis of the left lung base are primary physical signs of pancreatic pseudocyst. The principal differential diagnosis is upper abdominal neoplasm, particularly of the pancreas. **(REF. 1, p. 736)**

145. E. All of the items listed are actions of pure gastrin. Pancreozymin and cholecystokinin possess the same terminal tetrapeptide as gastrin and may explain extragastric effects of gastrin. **(REF. 1, p. 638)**

146. B. The gastric phase of gastric secretion encompasses antral gastrin secretion in response to local antral stimuli such as distention or alkali, and activation of local cholinergic reflexes. (REF. 1, p. 638)

147. A. A moderate to marked increase in the SGOT is not associated with cholestatic jaundice. Laboratory tests alone may not permit differentiation of intrahepatic from extrahepatic cholestasis. (REF. 1, p. 755)

148. D. In marked obstruction due to peptic ulcer, anorexia, nausea, and fullness after eating are the most frequent symptoms. An elevated hematocrit may also be present. (REF. 1, p. 652)

149. E. All the disorders listed are associated with protein-losing enteropathy. Intravenous administration of ^{125}I-labeled albumen may show up to a 40% loss in the GI tract in this condition. (REF. 1, p. 702)

150. E. The colon and rectum are supplied by all of the nerves and fibers listed. The functional significance of the sympathetic supply to the lower part of the intestine is unclear. (REF. 1, p. 1306)

151. A. Bile salts are good detergents, with polar and nonpolar groups that help dissolve fatty acids. Bile salts also form micelles and shift the pH optimum of lipases. (REF. 1, p. 679)

152. A. Acute necrotizing enterocolitis occurs in patients prepared for GI surgery with antibiotics or in liver disease patients on neomycin. Streptococcal invasion is not a characteristic of acute necrotizing enterocolitis. (REF. 1, p. 1497)

153. C. Black or "coffee-grounds" vomitus usually indicates bleeding proximal to the jejunum and vomiting several hours after bleeding. One must also consider swallowed blood from epistaxis, hemoptysis, dental extractions, and tonsillectomy. (REF. 1, p. 637)

Diseases of the Digestive System / 55

154. C. The patient is typically a middle-aged woman with itching, jaundice, steatorrhea, marked hepatomegaly, and elevated serum lipids. **(REF.** 1, p. 801**)**

155. B. The small bowel mucosal biopsy is abnormal in sprue, Whipple's disease, abetalipoproteinemia and agammaglobulinemia. **(REF.** 1, p. 694**)**

156. A. In addition to the first three signs listed, abnormal puddling of barium and fistulous tracts are other helpful x-ray signs of ileitis. **(REF.** 1, p. 711**)**

157. B. Fixation of the bowel wall by a tumor may produce volvulus, most frequently in the sigmoid colon. **(REF.** 1, p. 726**)**

3. Diseases of the Respiratory System

DIRECTIONS: Each of the questions or incomplete statements below is followed by five suggested answers or completions. Select the **one** that is **best** in each case.

158. In primary pulmonary hypertension the disease process involves
    A. small pulmonary arteries
    B. large pulmonary arteries
    C. pulmonary capillaries
    D. fibrosis of the alveolar wall
    E. organic cardiac disease

159. Management of aspiration pneumonia includes all of the following EXCEPT
    A. antibiotics
    B. steroids
    C. oxygen
    D. sedation
    E. bronchoscopy

160. The hallmark of generalized obstructive disease is reduced
    A. vital capacity
    B. timed vital capacity
    C. arterial oxygen saturation
    D. tidal volume
    E. residual volume

161. Diffuse nodular fibrosis of the lung with "eggshell" calcification of lymph nodes indicates
    A. cigarette smoking
    B. lung cancer
    C. asbestosis
    D. hypersensitivity pneumonitis
    E. silicosis

162. Which one of the following is characteristic of farmer's lung?
    A. Symptoms appear a few days after exposure
    B. It is caused by exposure to oxides of nitrogen
    C. It is usually followed by complete recovery
    D. It usually progresses to diffuse fibrosis
    E. It usually progresses to diffuse obstructive emphysema

163. Hypoventilation associated with depression of the respiratory center causes
    A. hypoxia and hypocapnia
    B. hypoxia and hypercapnia
    C. normal oxygen tension and hypercapnia
    D. hypoxia and normal CO_2 tension
    E. none of the above

164. Etiologic studies indicate that obstructive pulmonary emphysema is usually
    A. caused by bronchial asthma
    B. preceded by bronchitis
    C. due to childhood mucoviscidosis
    D. due to elastic tissue degeneration
    E. a forerunner of pulmonary carcinoma

165. Which of the following is seen in restrictive pulmonary diseases?
    A. Elevated arterial CO_2 tension
    B. Low alveolar CO_2 tension
    C. Respiratory alkalosis
    D. Hypocapnia
    E. None of the above

58 / Diseases of the Respiratory System

166. The syndrome of carbon dioxide narcosis
    A. occurs only with CO_2 inhalation
    B. does not occur in obstructive lung disease
    C. does not occur in restrictive lung disease
    D. may worsen with oxygen administration
    E. occurs with chronic hypocapnia

167. Characteristics of the primary focus of tuberculosis in the lung usually include all of the following EXCEPT
    A. initially exudative
    B. spread to local lymph nodes
    C. usually near the pleura
    D. noncaseation
    E. located in the lower part of the upper lobe

168. Dilatation of large bronchi with destruction of bronchial wall is seen in
    A. bronchiectasis
    B. emphysema
    C. pneumoconiosis
    D. bullae
    E. asthma

169. Pulmonary infiltrates with eosinophilia are seen in all of the following EXCEPT
    A. ascaris infestation
    B. malaria
    C. polyarteritis
    D. bronchial asthma
    E. penicillin sensitivity

170. Hypercapnia at rest in most individuals is most indicative of
    A. ventilation-perfusion ratio inequality
    B. right-to-left shunt
    C. impaired diffusion
    D. hypoventilation
    E. carbon monoxide poisoning

Diseases of the Respiratory System / 59

171. The volume of fresh gas entering the alveoli each minute is known as
    A. dead space
    B. diffusing capacity
    C. alveolar ventilation
    D. ventilation perfusion
    E. compliance

172. The most common cause of paresis or paralysis of the diaphragm due to phrenic nerve involvement is
    A. whiplash injury
    B. thyroid surgery
    C. mediastinitis
    D. tumor invasion
    E. adjacent pleural scarring

173. The most common primary posterior mediastinal tumor is
    A. lipoma
    B. neurogenic tumor
    C. esophageal cyst
    D. fibroma
    E. bronchogenic cyst

174. Familial emphysema may be associated with
    A. alpha-1-antitrypsin deficiency
    B. beta-glycosidase deficiency
    C. glucose-6-phosphatase deficiency
    D. glucocerebrosidase deficiency
    E. growth hormone deficiency

175. Features of lipid pneumonia can include all of the following EXCEPT
    A. mineral oil ingestion
    B. fat-laden macrophages
    C. bilateral lower lobe involvement
    D. paraffinoma
    E. hilar adenopathy

176. A patient with hypoxemia, hypercapnia, and polycythemia is able to restore his blood gases to normal by voluntary hyperventilation. The primary pathology is likely to be located in the
    A. cerebral cortex
    B. bone marrow
    C. ventricular septum
    D. medullary respiratory center
    E. cerebellum

177. Clubbing without cyanosis may be seen in all of the following EXCEPT
    A. subacute bacterial endocarditis
    B. ulcerative colitis
    C. occupational effect
    D. well-compensated mitral stenosis
    E. some healthy persons

DIRECTIONS: Each group of questions below consists of a list of lettered headings followed by a list of numbered words, phrases or statements. For **each** numbered word, phrase or statement, select the **one** lettered heading that is most closely associated with it. Each lettered heading may be selected once, more than once, or not at all.

    A. Epidermoid carcinoma
    B. Adenocarcinoma
    C. Large cell carcinoma
    D. Small cell carcinoma
    E. Bronchiolo-alveolar carcinoma

178. The most common type of lung cancer associated with hypercalcemia

179. Most responsive to cytotoxic chemotherapy

180. Overall best survival by natural history or after surgery

181. Most commonly associated with ectopic endocrine syndromes

182. This variety of lung cancer is frequently diffuse at presentation and may be associated with profuse sputum production

---

DIRECTIONS: Each set of lettered headings below is followed by a list of numbered words or phrases. For each numbered word or phrase select
    A if the item is associated with (A) *only,*
    B if the item is associated with (B) *only,*
    C if the item is associated with *both* (A) *and* (B),
    D if the item is associated with *neither* (A) *nor* (B).

    A. Silicosis
    B. Asbestosis
    C. Both
    D. Neither

183. The majority of cases are occupation-related

184. Most cases are chronic requiring many years of repeated exposure

185. As the disease progresses, pleural plaques are seen on chest x-ray

186. Hilar lymph nodes may develop "eggshell" calcifications

187. The pathologic hallmark of exposure is ferruginous bodies

62 / Diseases of the Respiratory System

DIRECTIONS: For each of the questions or incomplete statements below, **one** or **more** of the answers or completions given is correct. Select
- A if only *1, 2 and 3* are correct,
- B if only *1 and 3* are correct,
- C if only *2 and 4* are correct,
- D if only *4* is correct,
- E if *all* are correct.

188. Pathophysiologic features of obstructive pulmonary emphysema include
    1. increased functional residual capacity
    2. increased residual volume
    3. increased airway resistance
    4. reduced maximal breathing capacity

189. A restrictive pulmonary disease pattern can occur in
    1. myasthenia gravis
    2. kyphoscoliosis
    3. rheumatoid spondylitis
    4. pleural fibrosis

190. Systemic syndromes associated with lung cancer include
    1. inappropriate ADH secretion
    2. acanthosis nigricans
    3. Cushing's syndrome
    4. leukemoid reaction

191. Carbon dioxide retention is commonly seen in
    1. ventilation-perfusion ratio inequality
    2. impaired diffusion syndromes
    3. hypoventilation
    4. right-to-left shunt

192. The diagnosis of asbestosis is aided by finding
    1. bilateral pleural calcifications
    2. crackling basal rales
    3. clubbing of the fingers
    4. peritoneal mesothelioma

193. Symptoms of acute pulmonary thromboembolism include
    1. dyspnea
    2. syncope
    3. substernal pressure
    4. seizures

194. Prolonged hyperventilation syndrome may be associated with
    1. paresthesias
    2. low bicarbonate
    3. tetany
    4. palpitation

195. Pulmonary sarcoidosis may show which of the following types of physiologic features?
    1. Restrictive disease with no diffusion impairment
    2. Restrictive disease with diffusion impairment
    3. Increased airflow resistance
    4. No physiologic abnormalities

196. A 60-year-old man develops severe and rapidly progressive dyspnea associated with a diffuse pulmonary infiltrate on x-ray. Biopsy of the lung reveals carcinomatosis. Likely sites of origin are
    1. bronchogenic carcinoma
    2. carcinoma of the posterior nasopharynx
    3. carcinoma of the stomach
    4. basal cell carcinoma

197. The treatment of chronic airway obstruction includes
    1. cessation of smoking
    2. long-term steroids
    3. tetracycline for infection
    4. increased caloric intake

198. Causes of mediastinal emphysema include
    1. thoracocentesis
    2. apical tuberculosis
    3. tension pneumothorax
    4. pericarditis

Directions Summarized

A	B	C	D	E
1,2,3 only	1,3 only	2,4 only	4 only	All are correct

199. Restrictive respiratory disease is seen in
1. amyotropic lateral sclerosis
2. poliomyelitis
3. myasthenia gravis
4. myotonic dystrophy

200. Pulmonary infiltrations seen in early sarcoidosis
1. are usually associated with decreased arterial O_2 saturation
2. may resolve completely
3. usually progress to diffuse fibrosis
4. often respond to steroids

201. Hypoxemia while receiving 100% oxygen indicates
1. ventilation-perfusion ratio inequality
2. hypoventilation
3. impaired diffusion
4. right-to-left shunt

202. A 50-year-old man with severe kyphoscoliosis is most likely to have
1. enlarged overall lung volume
2. alveolar hyperventilation
3. left rather than right ventricular failure
4. recurrent pulmonary infections

203. Reduction of the ratio of forced expiratory volume to vital capacity (FEV/VC) is seen in
1. ankylosing spondylitis
2. Pickwickian syndrome
3. scleroderma of the chest wall
4. emphysema

Diseases of the Respiratory System / 65

DIRECTIONS: This section consists of situations, each followed by a series of questions. Study each situation, and select the **one** best answer to each question following it.

CASE 1 (Questions 204-208): A Negro female presents with mild dyspnea on exertion, arthralgia, fever, and erythema nodosum. Physical examination reveals hepatosplenomegaly, generalized lymphadenopathy, and corneal opacities. X-ray of the chest shows biliterally symmetrical hilar adenopathy.

204. The most likely diagnosis is
 A. Hodgkin's disease
 B. tuberculosis
 C. rheumatic fever
 D. sarcoidosis
 E. rheumatoid arthritis

205. All of the following laboratory results are likely to be present EXCEPT
 A. hyperglobulinemia
 B. hypocalcemia
 C. elevated sedimentation rate
 D. normal serum phosphorus
 E. mild anemia

206. Which of the following laboratory tests would be most likely to be positive?
 A. Tuberculin test
 B. Alcohol tolerance test
 C. Latex fixation
 D. Antistreptolysin-O (ASLO) titer
 E. Kveim test

207. The eye lesion is probably due to
 A. uveitis
 B. diabetic complications
 C. steroids
 D. congenital origin
 E. infectious infiltration

208. This disease is best treated with
   A. aspirin
   B. isoniazid and streptomycin
   C. steroids
   D. nitrogen mustard
   E. no therapy

CASE 2 (Questions 209-213): A 30-year-old male presents with a history of recurrent pneumonias and a chronic cough productive of foul-smelling, purulent sputum, occasionally blood-tinged, which is worse in the morning and on lying down. On physical examination the patient appears chronically ill with clubbing of the fingers. Wet inspiratory rales are heard at the lung bases posteriorly.

209. The most likely diagnosis is
   A. bronchiectasis
   B. chronic bronchitis
   C. disseminated pulmonary tuberculosis
   D. pulmonary neoplasm
   E. chronic obstructive emphysema

210. The most commonly involved area is likely to be the
   A. apical segment of the upper lobe
   B. posterior basal segments of the lower lobes
   C. lingula
   D. right middle lobe
   E. superior segments of the lower lobes

211. The most likely precursor of the above condition was
   A. bronchial asthma
   B. endobronchial tuberculosis
   C. pertussis
   D. bronchopneumonia
   E. influenza

Diseases of the Respiratory System / 67

212. The most important procedure necessary to define the extent of the disease would be
    A. tomography
    B. bronchoscopy
    C. bronchography
    D. open thoractomy
    E. gastric washings

213. Therapy for this disease might include
    A. antibiotics and postural drainage
    B. steroids
    C. radiotherapy
    D. aerosols
    E. isoniazid

CASE 3 (Questions 214-218): A 45-year-old bartender is admitted in a drowsy state, unable to give a history. Physical examination reveals a markedly obese, white male with a ruddy complexion, periodic respiration, cyanosis, and peripheral edema. His temperature is 102°F and his hematocrit is 55%.

214. The most likely diagnosis is
    A. alcoholic myocardiopathy
    B. hepatoma with secondary polycythemia
    C. pulmonary-cardiac failure associated with obesity
    D. polycythemia rubra vera associated with pneumonia
    E. acute alcoholic stupor associated with pneumonia

215. Blood gas determinations are likely to show arterial
    A. hypoxemia and hypercapnia
    B. hypoxemia and hypocapnia
    C. normal CO_2 and marked hypoxemia
    D. cyanosis only relative to hematocrit with normal O_2 tension and hypercapnia
    E. hyperoxemia and hypocapnia

68 / Diseases of the Respiratory System

216. Measurement of lung function is likely to show
    A. decrease of total lung capacity
    B. increased vital capacity
    C. normal expiratory reserve volume
    D. increased expiratory flow rate
    E. increased carbon dioxide exchange

217. Emergency treatment should include
    A. administration of 100% O_2 by mask
    B. intravenous saline given at 100 cc per hour
    C. pleural tap and culture of pleural fluid
    D. venesection with removal of 500 cc whole blood
    E. mechanical respiratory assistance

218. The best long-term therapy includes
    A. digitalis
    B. rapid weight loss
    C. prednisone
    D. radioactive phosphorus
    E. tetracycline

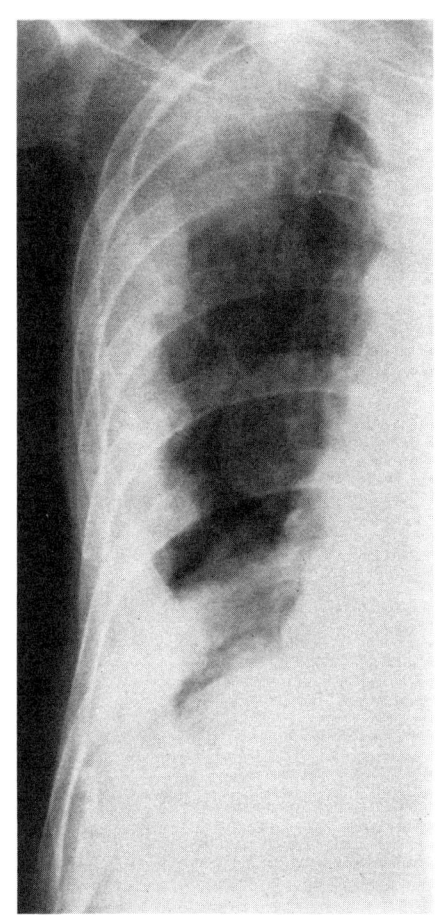

Figure 3.1

219. A 58-year-old steampipe worker had vague ache in the right chest and mild dyspnea of several months' duration. There was flatness on percussion of the right chest, associated with diminished breath sounds (Fig. 3.1). What is your diagnosis?
    A. Pleural metastases
    B. Paget's disease
    C. Mesothelioma and asbestosis
    D. Pleural effusion
    E. Multiple myeloma

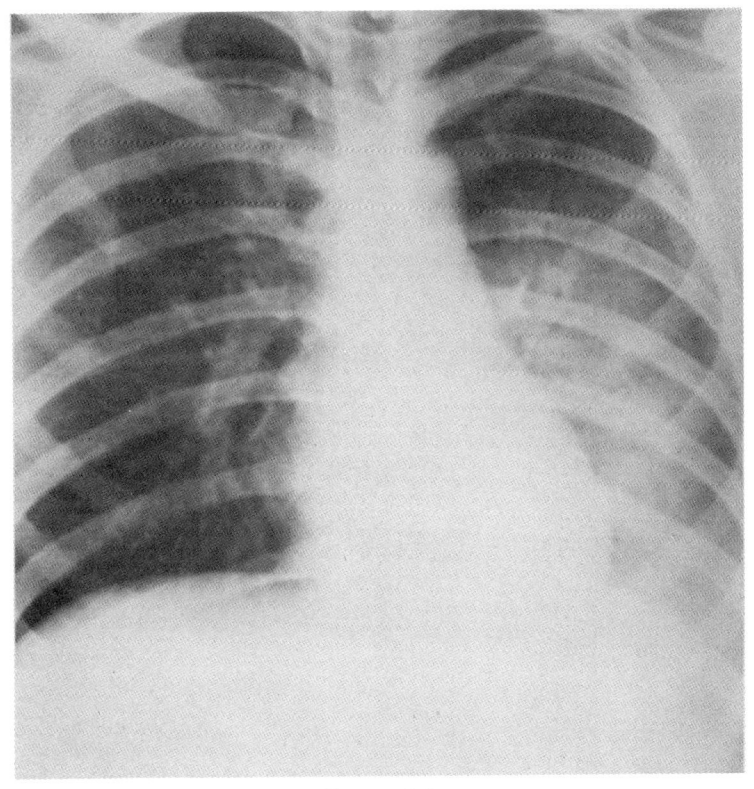

Figure 3.2

220. Cough with blood-tinged sputum, chills, and fever of two days' duration brought this 24-year-old man to the hospital. Physical findings revealed dullness and moist rales in the left lower chest (Fig. 3.2). What is your diagnosis?
    A. Pneumonia, left lower lobe
    B. Atelectasis, left lower lobe
    C. Pulmonary embolism
    D. Tuberculosis
    E. Sarcoidosis

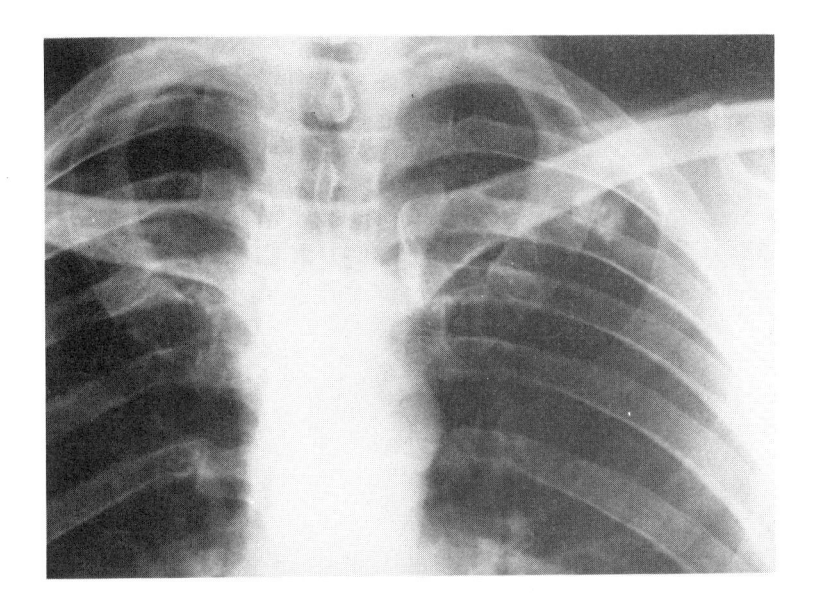

Figure 3.3

221. This is a close-up view of a chest x-ray from a 40-year-old man for insurance checkup (Fig. 3.3). What is your diagnosis?
    A. Hamartoma of the lung
    B. Tuberculous granuloma of the left apex
    C. Osteochondroma of the left fourth rib
    D. Bronchogenic carcinoma
    E. Pulmonary metastases

72 / Diseases of the Respiratory System

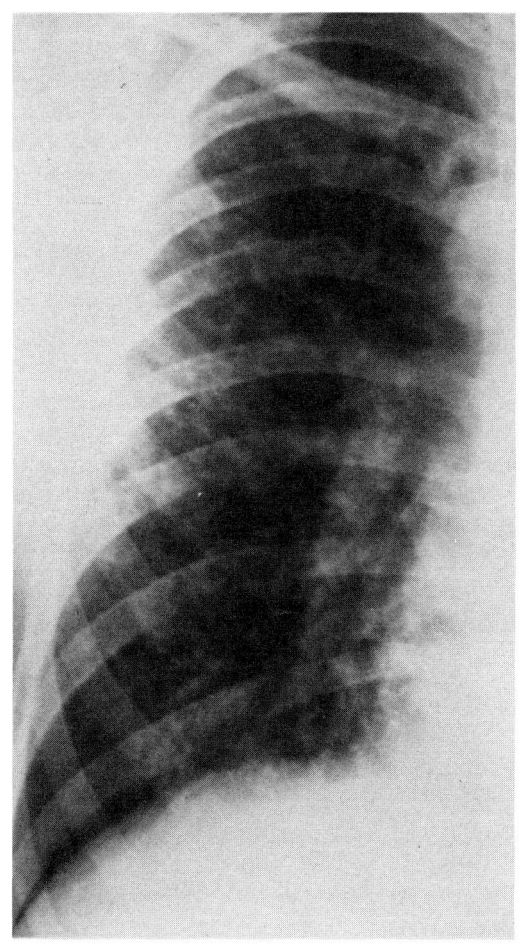

Figure 3.4

222. A 17-year-old male had slight tightness of the chest on heavy breathing, of two days' duration. He had pain in the left arm, which showed a lytic lesion on x-ray (Fig. 3.4). What is your diagnosis?
    A. Eosinophilic granuloma
    B. Cystic fibrosis
    C. Pulmonary metastases
    D. Bronchiectasis
    E. Tuberculosis

Pulmonary Function Studies

Chronic $PaCO_2$ mm Hg	35
Chronic PaO_2 mm Hg	70
Hematocrit %	35
Pulmonary Hypertension	
Rest	None
Exercise	Moderate
Elastic Recoil	Severly Decreased
Resistance	Normal
Diffusing Capacity	Decreased

223. The pulmonary function studies shown in the above chart are of a 65-year-old man with severe dyspnea and cough. The most likely diagnosis is
   A. emphysema
   B. lobar pneumonia
   C. chronic bronchitis
   D. acute bronchitis
   E. congestive heart failure

3. Diseases of the Respiratory System Answers and Comments

158. A. Small pulmonary arteries between 40 and 300 microns exhibit muscular hypertrophy and intimal hyperplasia. **(REF. 2, p. 1247)**

159. D. An acute inflammation of the lungs is produced by hydrochloric acid, and obstructive atelectasis results from inhaled solid material. **(REF. 2, p. 1223)**

160. B. In addition to reduced timed vital capacity, forced expiratory volume in one second (FEV_1) is also reduced and may be an early sign of generalized obstructive disease. **(REF. 2, p. 1235)**

161. E. In silicosis, lung function changes are variable and do not correlate well with x-ray changes. **(REF. 2, p. 1220)**

162. C. When exposure to moldy hay is stopped, symptoms and signs of farmer's lung all tend to abate and complete recovery usually follows. **(REF. 2, p. 1211)**

163. B. Hypoventilation associated with depression of the respiratory center causes hypoxia and hypercapnia. Causes of hypoxia and hypercapnia include drugs, anesthetics, central nervous system abnormalities, and idiopathic types. **(REF. 2, p. 1272)**

164. B. Bronchitis usually precedes obstructive pulmonary emphysema. This type of patient is often short and fat with a plethoric complexion and wet cough. **(REF. 2, p. 1235)**

165. A. Elevated CO_2 tension is seen in restrictive pulmonary diseases. Restrictive disease leads to hypoventilation with hypoxia and hypercapnia. Hypoxia is corrected with 100% oxygen. **(REF. 2, p. 1241)**

166. D. Administration of oxygen may worsen the syndrome

Diseases of the Respiratory System / 75

of carbon dioxide narcosis because the chief stimulus to ventilation is often hypoxia, and when this is suddenly relieved the ventilation may drop quickly. **(REF. 2, p. 1241)**

167. D. The typical reaction to primary TB includes epithelioid cell granuloma with caseation necrosis. **(REF. 2, p. 702)**

168. A. In bronchiectasis large bronchi, greater than 2 mm, are affected, and muscular and elastic components are destroyed. **(REF. 2, p. 1230)**

169. B. Etiology remains obscure in most cases of pulmonary eosinophilia, but infestation is often suspect. Malaria is not seen in these cases. **(REF. 2, p. 1210)**

170. D. Hypoventilation always causes both hypoxemia and hypercapnia. **(REF. 2, p. 1198)**

171. C. The alveolar ventilation is about 5 liters on the average. **(REF. 2, p. 1191)**

172. D. Phrenic nerve paralysis of the diaphragm produces upward displacement and paradoxic movement of the diaphragm with respiration and is most commonly caused by tumor invasion. **(REF. 2, p. 1260)**

173. B. Neurogenic tumor is the most common primary posterior mediastinal tumor. Other tumors include cysts, teratodermoids, thymomas, and lymphomas. **(REF. 2, p. 1269)**

174. A. Most normal persons have two M genes, but the Z gene is responsible for low production of alpha-1-antitrypsin, a condition associated with familial emphysema. **(REF. 2, p. 1236)**

175. E. Hilar adenopathy is not a feature of lipid pneumonia. The chest x-ray may show patchy or nodular lesions, particularly at the lung bases. **(REF. 2, p. 1215)**

176. D. The primary pathology is likely to be located in the

Diseases of the Respiratory System

medullary respiratory center. Cyanosis, especially when asleep, is caused by a combination of polycythemia and hypoxia. **(REF. 2, p. 1191)**

177. D. Clubbing without cyanosis is not seen in well-compensated mitral stenosis. Hypertrophic osteoarthropathy frequently occurs with digital clubbing but may precede clubbing or develop without it. **(REF. 2, p. 1261)**

178. A. Hypercalcemia may be due to metastatic destruction of bone, ectopic formation of parathyroid hormone, or formation of other osteolytic substances. **(REF. 1, p. 415)**

179. D. Combination chemotherapy has produced promising results in lung cancer, particularly of the small cell anaplastic type. Alkylating agents and anthracyclines are active amongst other agents. **(REF. 1, p. 418)**

180. A. The two-year survival of patients with epidermoid carcinoma is 46% for stage I and 40% for stage II. Adenocarcinoma is also associated with a relatively good stage I survival, but a much worse stage II survival. **(REF. 1, p. 418)**

181. D. The most commonly encountered syndromes are inappropriate antidiuretic hormone secretion, Cushing's syndrome, and gynecomastia. **(REF. 1, p. 415)**

182. E. Bronchiolo-alveolar carcinoma is a variety of adenocarcinoma but spreads in a diffuse pattern throughout the lungs. It is associated with a particularly poor prognosis. **(REF. 1, pp. 415, 418)**

183. C. Silicosis is seen in mining, stone cutting, sandblasting, and foundry work. Asbestosis is associated with mining, milling, shipyard work, and insulation work. **(REF. 1, pp. 399, 401)**

184. C. There is a rare acute form of silicosis which occurs in less than 5 years but most cases of both diseases are seen after 5 to 25 years of exposure. **(REF. 1, pp. 400, 401)**

Diseases of the Respiratory System / 77

185. B. Pleural plaques can best be seen on oblique views but care must be taken to differentiate true plaques from shadows produced by muscle attachments. **(REF. 1, p. 401)**

186. A. Silicotic nodules become calcified in the upper lung lobes, and hilar lymph nodes enlarge and develop thin lines of calcification. **(REF. 1, p. 400)**

187. B. These structures are 2 to 5 microns wide and 20 to 150 microns long. Although the core can occasionally be silicate particles, asbestos fibre is usually the cause. **(REF. 1, p. 401)**

188. E. In addition to all of the features listed, forced expiratory volume in one second is also reduced and vital capacity may be low. **(REF. 2, p. 1235)**

189. E. In all of these conditions there is alveolar hypoventilation, resulting in low Po_2 and elevated Pco_2. **(REF. 2, p. 1236)**

190. E. Syndromes are classified as metabolic, neuromuscular, connective tissue, dermatologic, and vascular. All of the systemic syndromes listed are associated with lung cancer. **(REF. 2, p. 1259)**

191. B. Carbon dioxide retention is seen in right-to-left shunt only with exercise and is uncommon in impaired diffusion syndromes. **(REF. 2, p. 1194)**

192. E. Asbestos slowly causes a diffuse pulmonary fibrosis after a long latent period. Its diagnosis is aided by finding all of the signs listed. **(REF. 2, p. 1219)**

193. A. In acute pulmonary thromboembolism, pleuritic chest pain and hemoptysis are present only when infarction has occurred, and seizures are not symptomatic. **(REF. 2, p. 1249)**

194. E. Prolonged hyperventilation syndrome may be associated with all of the conditions listed. The patient is often a

78 / Diseases of the Respiratory System

nervous, anxious woman who has other functional disturbances due to tension. (**REF.** 2, p. 1192)

195. E. Pulmonary sarcoidosis may show all of the features listed. Spontaneous permanent remissions are observed, but significant lung disease represents the major indication for treatment. (**REF.** 2, p. 1120)

196. B. Bronchogenic carcinoma and carcinoma of the stomach are the most likely. The triad of bronchoscopy, scalene lymph node biopsy, and cytologic smear is usually most helpful. (**REF.** 2, p. 1259)

197. B. Treatment includes cessation of smoking and tetracycline. Some patients respond to steroids, but these are only used in strictly controlled circumstances. (**REF.** 2, p. 1235)

198. B. In addition to thoracocentesis and tension pneumothorax, mediastinal emphysema may result from traumatic perforation of the trachea or esophagus, rupture of the alveoli, or dissection of the retroperitoneum. (**REF.** 2, p. 1270)

199. E. Restrictive respiratory disease is seen in all of the conditions cited. Neuromuscular disorders are a common cause of hypoventilation. Others include thoracic cage abnormalities and medullary failure. (**REF.** 2, p. 1241)

200. C. In early sarcoidosis, pulmonary infiltration may resolve completely and often respond to steroids. Cough may be severe and incapacitating and may occur in paroxysms leading to vomiting. (**REF.** 2, p. 929)

201. D. Hypoxemia while receiving 100% oxygen indicates right-to-left shunt. Shunts permit circulation of blood that never passes through the ventilated lung. (**REF.** 2, p. 1191)

202. D. This patient is most likely to have recurrent pulmonary infections. Bony deformities of the chest can lead to respiratory failure with raised $P{CO_2}$. (**REF.** 2, p. 1273)

Diseases of the Respiratory System / 79

203. D. The vital capacity is reduced in emphysema, but the FEV$_1$ is grossly reduced because of high airway resistance. **(REF.** 2, p. 1235)

204. D. Sarcoidosis is the most likely diagnosis. Granulomatous inflammatory changes of sarcoidosis may occur in almost any organ. **(REF.** 2, p. 928)

205. B. Hypocalcemia is not a laboratory result. Hypercalcemia infrequently occurs, but may result from increased intestinal absorption of calcium. **(REF.** 2, p. 930)

206. E. The Kveim test requires six weeks' incubation and must be biopsied to be interpreted. **(REF.** 2, p. 931)

207. A. Acute granulomatous uveitis may be the initial manifestation of sarcoidosis. **(REF.** 2, p. 929)

208. C. Relatively asymptomatic patients often require no treatment. Steroids are used with ocular, central nervous system, or other serious complications. **(REF.** 2, p. 931)

209. A. Bronchiectasis is defined as a permanent abnormal dilatation of large bronchi, due to destruction of the wall. **(REF.** 2, p. 1230)

210. B. The posterior basal segments of the lower lobes are likely to be the most commonly involved area. True bronchiectasis is not reversible, but reversible conditions such as tracheobronchitis may simulate it. **(REF.** 2, p. 1230)

211. D. Bronchopneumonia was the most likely precursor of the bronchiectasis. Hereditary, congenital, or mechanical factors usually predispose to recurrent infection. **(REF.** 2, p. 1230)

212. C. Bronchography is the most important procedure necessary in defining the extent of bronchiectasis. Occasionally, advanced cases of saccular bronchiectasis can be diagnosed by routine chest x-ray. **(REF.** 2, p. 1231)

213. A. Antibiotics and postural drainage might be included in therapy. The choice of antimicrobial agents is guided by the sputum culture, but ampicillin and tetracycline are used if normal flora are found. **(REF. 2, p. 1232)**

214. C. Pulmonary-cardiac failure associated with obesity is the most likely diagnosis. The obesity may be present for years, but in some cases rapid weight gain has been described. **(REF. 2, p. 1273)**

215. A. Arterial hypoxemia and hypercapnea are likely to show in blood gas determinations. P_{CO_2} may be as high as 70 mm of mercury. The ventilatory response to inhaled CO_2 is generally decreased. **(REF. 2, p. 1274)**

216. A. Measurement of lung function is likely to show a decrease of total lung capacity. The expiratory reserve volume and vital capacity are reduced as is the chest wall compliance. **(REF. 2, p. 1272)**

217. E. Mechanical respiratory assistance should be included in emergency treatment. P_{O_2} levels below 40 mmHg may be associated with arrhythmias, impaired cardiac and cerebral function, and liver and kidney impairment. **(REF. 2, p. 1274)**

218. B. Dramatic improvement in all indices occurs with weight loss, and signs of heart failure may disappear. **(REF. 2, p. 1274)**

219. C. There is moderate pleural thickening with scalloped margins from apex to base. There is a similar finding in the mediastinal and diaphragmatic pleura. Furthermore, there is a plaque of pleural calcification in the base. The association of asbestosis with mesothelioma has long been known. As the neoplasma progresses, it may envelop the thorax. **(REF. 2, pp. 1265, 1269)**

220. A. The diagnosis is pneumonia. There is consolidation of the left lower lobe. The increased density, presence of air bronchogram, and the silhouetting of the left diaphragm point

Diseases of the Respiratory System / 81

to a parenchymal lesion. Pneumococcal infection, as in this patient, is still the most common etiology, although other bacterial infections such as *Klebsiella*, streptococcus, or staphylococcus are often encountered. Viral and arthropod-borne diseases are also seen. (**REF. 2, p. 604**)

221. B. There is a calcified nodule in the left apex. Obviously, a calcified tuberculous granuloma is the most common lesion. This may be from reinfection tuberculosis, where its preference for the apico-posterior segment is well known. It is also possible that it may be a calcified Ghon's lesion. (**REF. 2, pp. 702-705**)

222. A. Eosinophilic granuloma is the diagnosis. There is a coarse, reticular pattern in the whole lung—somewhat more prominent in the upper lobes—suggesting a honeycomb appearance. It is the density here which is abnormal and not the lucency. (**REF. 2, p. 1582**)

223. A. Because of the maintained increase in minute volume and the maintenance of arterial Pao_2, patients with emphysema are referred to as "pink puffers." (**REF. 2, p. 1239**)

4. Diseases of the Cardiovascular System

DIRECTIONS: Each of the questions or incomplete statements below is followed by five suggested answers or completions. Select the **one** that is **best** in each case.

224. Wenckebach's typed AV block is recognized by
    A. progressive P-Q shortening
    B. progressive lengthening of the P-R interval
    C. tachycardia
    D. dropped beat after P-Q lengthening
    E. fixed 2:1 block

225. Which one of the following is an electrocardiographic sign of hypercalcemia?
    A. Shortened P-R interval
    B. Lengthened P-R interval
    C. Lengthened Q-U interval
    D. Shortening of the Q-T interval
    E. Shortening of the Q-U interval

226. A pacemaker that functions when the heart rate falls below a present interval is called
    A. asynchronous
    B. atrial synchronous
    C. ventricular synchronous
    D. ventricular standby
    E. atrial sequential

227. The electrocardiographic signs of pulmonary embolism include all of the following EXCEPT
 A. a deep S_1
 B. depressed S-T in leads I and II
 C. prominent Q_3 and inversion of T_3
 D. left axis deviation
 E. clockwise rotation in the precordial leads

228. Angina pectoris and syncope are most likely to be associated with
 A. mitral stenosis
 B. mitral insufficiency
 C. aortic stenosis
 D. aortic insufficiency
 E. tricuspid stenosis

229. Bacterial endocarditis may include all of the following complications EXCEPT
 A. normocytic anemia
 B. sudden peripheral gangrene
 C. peripheral neuropathy
 D. hematuria
 E. aortic insufficiency

230. The third heart sound may be heard in all of the following EXCEPT
 A. children
 B. young adults with anemia
 C. mitral regurgitation
 D. mitral stenosis
 E. tricuspid regurgitation

231. Chest pain and friction rub three days after admission to a coronary care unit probably indicate
 A. misdiagnosis of infarction
 B. chest trauma
 C. viral infection
 D. transmural infarction
 E. dissecting aneurysm

232. The effect of calcium ions on the myocardium can best be described as
    A. positively inotropic
    B. negatively inotropic
    C. positively chronotropic
    D. negatively chronotropic
    E. excitation-contraction uncoupling

233. Which of the following is seen as a manifestation of myxedema heart disease?
    A. High output heart failure
    B. Pericardial effusion
    C. Decreased incidence of coronary artery disease
    D. Higher incidence of atrial arrhythmias
    E. Decreased arteriovenous oxygen difference

234. The temporary or standby pacemaker may be indicated in acute myocardial infarction with all of the following EXCEPT
    A. persistent bradycardia
    B. inferior infarction and block
    C. pericardial rub and tachycardia
    D. alternating right and left bundle-branch block
    E. Mobitz type 2 block

235. Which of the following is associated with an increased intensity of the pulmonic second heart sound?
    A. Pulmonary stenosis
    B. Aortic stenosis
    C. Myocardial infarction
    D. Pulmonary hypertension
    E. Systemic hypertension

236. Sympathetic stimulation to the heart
    A. is transmitted by acetylcholine
    B. is the dominant autonomic influence on heart rate
    C. is mediated by release of norepinephrine
    D. bypasses the cardiac plexus
    E. travels through the vagus nerve

237. A patient with a regular heart beat at a rate of 170 per minute that abruptly changes to 75 per minute after applying carotid sinus pressure most likely has
    A. sinus tachycardia
    B. paroxysmal atrial fibrillation
    C. paroxysmal atrial flutter
    D. paroxysmal atrial tachycardia
    E. paroxysmal ventricular tachycardia

238. Which of the following is NOT an electrocardiographic finding of acute myocarditis?
    A. Prolonged P-R interval
    B. S-T segment depressions
    C. Inverted T waves
    D. S-T segment elevations
    E. Significant Q waves

239. Angina pectoris, in the absence of coronary artery disease, occurs most frequently with
    A. mitral stenosis
    B. mitral insufficiency
    C. pulmonary stenosis
    D. aortic stenosis
    E. aortic insufficiency

240. In aortic stenosis the second aortic sound at the base is characteristically
    A. accentuated
    B. diminished
    C. normal in character
    D. widely split due to delayed ventricular ejection
    E. shows fixed splitting

241. Atrioventricular dissociation is defined as
    A. surgical removal of an atrium
    B. independent beating of atria and ventricles
    C. congenital absence of atrial and ventricular septa
    D. oxygen differential between chambers
    E. heart rate under 60 beats per minute

86 / Diseases of the Cardiovascular System

242. Giant a waves in the venous pulse are associated with all of the following EXCEPT
    A. patent ductus arteriosus
    B. tricuspid atresia
    C. pulmonary stenosis
    D. acute pulmonary embolism
    E. tricuspid stenosis

243. Reversed splitting of the second heart sound is associated with all of the following EXCEPT
    A. left bundle-branch block
    B. disappearance of split on inspiration
    C. prolongation of right ventricular systole
    D. prolongation of left ventricular systole
    E. delayed activation of the left ventricle

244. Of the following congenital lesions, which is the most frequently complicated by subacute bacterial endocarditis (SBE)?
    A. Ventricular septal defects
    B. Atrial septal defects
    C. Transposition of the great vessels
    D. Aortic stenosis
    E. Congenital mitral insufficiency

245. Atrial flutter with 2:1 block would most likely demonstrate
    A. a ventricular rate of 300/min
    B. an atrial rate of 300/min
    C. an atrial rate of 150/min
    D. the same atrial and ventricular rates
    E. a ventricular rate of 300/min and an atrial rate of 150/min

246. The most common cause of death from subacute bacterial endocarditis is
    A. myocardial abscesses
    B. cerebral abscesses
    C. rupture of the involved valve
    D. generalized toxemia
    E. congestive heart failure

247. EKG changes after myocardial infarction reflect changes in initial forces away from the infarct area, because a different sequence of depolarization is produced in the
    A. ventricle
    B. SA node
    C. AV node
    D. right atrium
    E. aorta

248. The most common primary cardiac tumor is a
    A. myxoma
    B. sarcoma
    C. rhabdomyoma
    D. fibroma
    E. lipoma

249. Exercise electrocardiography
    A. is an invasive procedure
    B. is contraindicated in patients over 65
    C. detects latent disease
    D. has a morbidity of approximately 5%
    E. is used in pulmonary embolism

250. The valves most commonly involved in rheumatic heart disease are
    A. mitral and tricuspid
    B. tricuspid and pulmonary
    C. pulmonary and aortic
    D. mitral and pulmonary
    E. mitral and aortic

88 / Diseases of the Cardiovascular System

251. Cardiac catheterization
   A. is contraindicated in the presence of cyanosis
   B. is considered noninvasive
   C. is generally performed with cardiopulmonary bypass
   D. may be an electrical hazard
   E. requires carotid artery puncture

252. Pericarditis is known to occur with each of the following diseases EXCEPT
   A. rheumatic fever
   B. tuberculosis
   C. pneumonia
   D. myocardial infarction
   E. scarlet fever

253. In a patient with mitral regurgitation, dye injected into the left ventricle during an angiogram procedure would show
   A. dye rapidly appearing in the right atrium, right ventricle, and the pulmonary artery
   B. dye slowly appearing in the left ventricle
   C. dye rapidly appearing in the lungs
   D. dye rapidly appearing in the left atrium, left ventricle, and the aorta
   E. none of the above

254. During cardiac catheterization the pulmonary "wedged" capillary pressure is an approximation of pressure in the
   A. pulmonary artery
   B. pulmonary vein
   C. left atrium
   D. right atrium
   E. vena cava

Diseases of the Cardiovascular System / 89

255. In atrial septal defects
   A. pulmonary blood flow is greater than systemic blood flow
   B. pulmonary blood flow is less than systemic blood flow
   C. pulmonary blood flow is equal to systemic blood flow
   D. the left ventricle is enlarged
   E. the systemic blood pressure is elevated

256. Echocardiography is useful in the diagnosis of all of the following EXCEPT
   A. mitral stenosis
   B. coarctation of the aorta
   C. muscular subaortic stenosis
   D. atrial septal defect
   E. prosthetic valve dysfunction

257. A rapidly rising forceful pulse which collapses quickly is seen in which of the following lesions?
   A. Mitral stenosis
   B. Mitral regurgitation
   C. Aortic stenosis
   D. Aortic regurgitation
   E. Coarctation of the aorta

258. The most common cause of failure of the right ventricle is
   A. pulmonary embolus
   B. mitral stenosis
   C. pulmonary hypertension
   D. congenital heart disease
   E. failure of the left ventricle

90 / Diseases of the Cardiovascular System

259. Mitral stenosis may be associated with all of the following clinical symptoms EXCEPT
   A. angina pectoris
   B. hoarseness
   C. cough
   D. hemoptysis
   E. nausea and vomiting

260. Digitalis is indicated in all of the following EXCEPT
   A. acute myocardial infarction
   B. atrial fibrillation
   C. atrial flutter
   D. congestive heart failure with regular sinus rhythm
   E. congestive heart failure with atrial fibrillation

261. The development of paroxysmal atrial tachycardia in a patient on digitalis indicates
   A. an increase in digitalis dose
   B. complete cessation of digitalis
   C. withdrawal of digitalis for one dose
   D. no change in digitalis, but other medication should be given
   E. none of the above

262. Chronic constrictive pericarditis is found in association with all of the following EXCEPT
   A. rheumatic fever
   B. tuberculosis
   C. unknown cause
   D. previous acute pericarditis
   E. neoplastic involvement of the pericardium

263. Digitalis given in atrial flutter frequently causes
   A. atrial asystole
   B. atrial bigeminy
   C. atrial tachycardia
   D. paroxysmal atrial tachycardia with block
   E. atrial fibrillation

264. A regular tachycardia may be any of the following EXCEPT
    A. sinus tachycardia
    B. atrial flutter
    C. nodal tachycardia
    D. atrial fibrillation
    E. ventricular tachycardia

265. All of the following may lead to some fluid retention in heart failure EXCEPT
    A. increased renin
    B. increased aldosterone
    C. increased estrogen
    D. increased growth hormone
    E. increased vasopressin

DIRECTIONS: Each group of questions below consists of a list of lettered headings followed by a list of numbered words, phrases or statements. For **each** numbered word, phrase or statement, select the **one** lettered heading that is most closely associated with it. Each lettered heading may be selected once, more than once, or not at all.

A. Atrial rate of 100 to 150 per minute
B. Atrial rate below 60 per minute
C. Atrial rate three times as fast as the ventricular rate
D. Ventricular rate of 250 per minute
E. Atrial rate of approximately 300 per minute
F. Atrial rate over 400 per minute
G. Ventricular rate below 40 per minute
H. Atrial rate of 140 to 220 per minute

266. Paroxysmal atrial tachycardia

267. Atrial flutter with 2:1 block

268. Atrial fibrillation

269. Ventricular flutter

270. Complete heart block

    A. Mitral stenosis
    B. Acute rheumatic fever
    C. Pericardial effusion
    D. Hyperparathyroidism
    E. Wolff-Parkinson-White syndrome
    F. Hypokalemia
    G. Hyperkalemia
    H. Aortic stenosis

271. Broad-notched P wave

272. Prolonged P-R interval

273. Short P-R interval

274. Short Q-T interval

275. Low-voltage QRS complexes

DIRECTIONS: Each set of lettered headings below is followed by a list of numbered words or phrases. For each numbered word or phrase select
    A if the item is associated with (A) *only,*
    B if the item is associated with (B) *only,*
    C if the item is associated with *both* (A) *and* (B),
    D if the item is associated with *neither* (A) *nor* (B).

    A. Acute pericarditis
    B. Anterior wall myocardial infarction
    C. Both
    D. Neither

276. Severe anterior chest pain is a presenting symptom

277. A characteristic physical finding is a pericardial friction rub

278. On the electrocardiogram, acutely elevated ST segments are usually seen

279. Elevation of myocardial enzymes is seen

    A. Propranolol
    B. Verapamil
    C. Both
    D. Neither

280. Well absorbed from the gastrointestinal tract with useful bioavailability

281. The effects on the heart result in a prominent negative inotropic effect

282. Treatment of choice in paroxysmal AV junctional tachycardias

283. Mechanism of action is calcium blockade

    A. Sick sinus syndrome
    B. Second-degree heart block
    C. Both
    D. Neither

284. Recognized by the absence of expected sinus P waves

285. The P-R interval undergoes gradual prolongation prior to block of an atrial impulse

286. P waves block suddenly and there is a bundle-branch block pattern

287. Digitalis is used if bradycardia leads to heart failure

94 / Diseases of the Cardiovascular System

DIRECTIONS: For each of the questions or incomplete statements below, **one** or **more** of the answers or completions given is correct. Select
- A if only *1, 2 and 3* are correct,
- B if only *1 and 3* are correct,
- C if only *2 and 4* are correct,
- D if only *4* is correct,
- E if *all* are correct.

288. Which of the following electrocardiographic signs may be seen in the presence of a ventricular aneurysm?
    1. Small R_1, deep S_2 and S_3
    2. RS-T depressions in V_5 and V_6
    3. Inversion of T waves in at least three precordial leads
    4. Presence of an rS in aVL

289. X-ray examination of the heart in aortic stenosis is likely to reveal
    1. right ventricular dilatation
    2. dilatation of the proxmial ascending aorta
    3. left atrial hypertrophy
    4. normal overall cardiac size

290. A pulsatile liver may be caused by
    1. tricuspid insufficiency
    2. aortic insufficiency
    3. tricuspid stenosis
    4. aortic stenosis

291. Blood pressure in the arms may differ significantly from pressure in the legs in the presence of
    1. coarctation of the aorta
    2. aortic insufficiency
    3. aortic occlusive disease
    4. normal children over 2 years old

292. The electrocardiographic signs of left ventricular hypertrophy include
    1. left axis deviation
    2. counterclockwise rotation of the electrical axis
    3. high voltage of the QRS complex in V_5 and V_6
    4. rsR' pattern in V_1

293. Which of the following occur in the presence of untreated, uncomplicated congestive heart failure?
    1. Increased urinary sodium content
    2. High urinary specific gravity
    3. Increased urinary chloride content
    4. Albuminuria

294. Which of the following electrocardiographic signs may be seen in the presence of acute pericarditis?
    1. S-T segment elevations without reciprocal depressions
    2. A normal electrocardiogram
    3. T wave inversions
    4. Significant Q waves

295. Cardiac findings secondary to hyperthyroid heart disease may include
    1. prolonged circulation time
    2. decreased cardiac output
    3. pericardial effusion
    4. paroxysmal atrial fibrillation

296. In atrial fibrillation, digitalis slows the ventricular rate by
    1. direct vagal stimulation
    2. depression of atrioventricular conduction in the AV node
    3. increasing ventricular contractility
    4. depressant action on the ventricular myocardial tissue

Directions Summarized				
A	B	C	D	E
1,2,3 only	1,3 only	2,4 only	4 only	All are correct

297. Objective end points for maximal exercise testing include
    1. supraventricular tachycardia
    2. ventricular tachycardia
    3. clammy skin
    4. systolic pressure greater than 140

298. In the presence of atrial fibrillation the ventricular rate will be regular if there is
    1. complete heart block
    2. advanced heart block
    3. ventricular tachycardia
    4. left bundle-branch block

299. Type II hyperlipoproteinemia may be secondary to
    1. myxedema
    2. nephrosis
    3. obstructive liver disease
    4. hyperthyroidism

300. The development of clinical symptomatology from a pericardial effusion depends on the
    1. quantity of effusion
    2. specific gravity
    3. rate of development of the effusion
    4. presence or absence of blood in the fluid

301. Diagnostic evaluation of patients with diastolic hypertension should include
    1. intravenous pyelogram
    2. chest x-ray
    3. serum potassium
    4. family history

Diseases of the Cardiovascular System / 97

DIRECTIONS: This section consists of situations, each followed by a series of questions. Study each situation, and select the **one** best answer to each question following it.

CASE 1 (Questions 302–306): A 36-year-old male is seen because of palpitations. He admits to precordial discomfort, weakness, and anxiety. The pulse is 160. The blood pressure is 100/70. The heart sounds are normal. Carotid sinus pressure changes the rate to 80, but when released the pulse rate returns to 160.

302. The most likely diagnosis is
 A. atrial flutter with 2:1 block
 B. paroxysmal atrial tachycardia with 2:1 block
 C. sinus arrhythmia
 D. atrial fibrillation
 E. nodal tachycardia

303. Prior to the use of drugs, which of the following procedures were helpful in converting the above to a sinus rhythm?
 A. Carotid sinus pressure
 B. Gagging procedures
 C. Valsalva's maneuver
 D. Eyeball compression
 E. None of the above

304. The drug of choice in treatment is
 A. digitalis
 B. Mecholyl
 C. aminophylline
 D. ephedrine
 E. atropine

98 / Diseases of the Cardiovascular System

305. The tachycardia is commonly associated with all of the following EXCEPT
  A. hypertensive disease
  B. rheumatic heart disease
  C. syphilitic heart disease
  D. coronary disease
  E. hyperthyroidism

306. The common complications of the arrhythmia include all of the following EXCEPT
  A. right heart failure
  B. peripheral arterial embolization
  C. syncope
  D. left heart failure
  E. pericarditis

CASE 2 (Questions 307-311): A 54-year-old female presents with dull precordial chest pain, dyspnea, and orthopnea of two weeks' duration. Physical examination reveals muffled heart sounds and diminution of pulse pressure by 25 mm Hg during inspiration.

307. The most likely diagnosis is
  A. myocardial infarction
  B. pericarditis with effusion
  C. emphysema with right heart failure
  D. rapid atrial fibrillation
  E. superior vena cava syndrome

308. Possible associated diseases include all of the following EXCEPT
  A. myocardial infarction
  B. tuberculosis
  C. uremia
  D. disseminated lupus erythematosus
  E. hyperthyroidism

309. Other physical signs may include all of the following EXCEPT
    A. giant a waves in the neck
    B. a to-and-fro scratching sound over the heart
    C. increased cardiac dullness to percussion
    D. dullness to percussion below the angle of the left scapula
    E. enlargement of the liver

310. In acute pericarditis the most consistent and significant electrocardiographic alteration is
    A. depression of the S-T segment in the precordial leads
    B. elevation of the S-T segment in the standard leads
    C. tall, peaked T waves
    D. prolongation of the Q-T interval
    E. shortening of the Q-T interval

311. If the patient suddenly becomes more dyspneic with an enlarging "heart" shadow on chest x-ray, the best treatment includes
    A. steroids
    B. digitalis
    C. furosemide or ethacrynic acid
    D. pericardiocentesis
    E. phlebotomy

CASE 3 (Questions 312–316): A 25-year-old man complains of left precordial chest pain that radiates to the left shoulder but not down the left arm. The pain is accentuated by inspiration and relieved by sitting up. The pain is accompanied by fever and chills. His blood pressure is 105/75, the pulse 110/min and regular, and the temperature is 102°F. Aside from the tachycardia there are no abnormal physical findings in the heart or lungs. The electrocardiogram shows S-T segment elevation in all leads except aVR and VI. On the third hospital day the blood pressure falls, the venous pressure rises, and the patient goes into congestive heart failure and shock.

Diseases of the Cardiovascular System

312. The most likely diagnosis is
    A. pulmonary infarction
    B. myocardial infarction
    C. pericarditis
    D. myocardial infarction with secondary pericarditis
    E. viral pneumonitis

313. The underlying etiologic factor is
    A. coronary atherosclerosis
    B. thrombophlebitis
    C. neoplasm
    D. unknown but probably viral
    E. an arteritis

314. The events of the third hospital day were probably caused by
    A. a second pulmonary embolus
    B. extension of a myocardial infarct
    C. cardiac tamponade
    D. secondary bacterial infection
    E. rupture of a chorda tendineae

315. The correct treatment on the third hospital day would be
    A. ligation of the inferior vena cava
    B. pericardiocentesis
    C. anticoagulation and pressor amines
    D. penicillin and oxygen
    E. coronary endarterectomy

316. The chest roentgenogram on the third hospital day would probably reveal
    A. a wedge-shaped area of consolidation in the left lung field and a left pleural effusion
    B. no abnormal findings
    C. a water-bottle heart
    D. patchy areas of consolidation in the left lung field
    E. hypervascular lung fields

Laboratory Investigations

Urinalysis	
pH	5.2
Albumin	negative to trace
Serum Na	140 meq/L
K	3.5 meq/L
Cl	100 meq/L
CO_2	25 meq/L
Creatinine	1.0 mg/100 ml
Fasting Sugar	90 mg/100 ml
Calcium	9.0 mg/100 ml
Uric acid	5.0 mg/100 ml

317. The laboratory results shown in the diagram above are obtained from the investigation of a 37-year-old black female who has a blood pressure at rest of 145/100 mm Hg. The most likely diagnosis is
A. Cushing's syndrome
B. primary aldosteronism
C. essential hypertension
D. pyelonephritis
E. bilateral renal artery stenosis

102 / Diseases of the Cardiovascular System

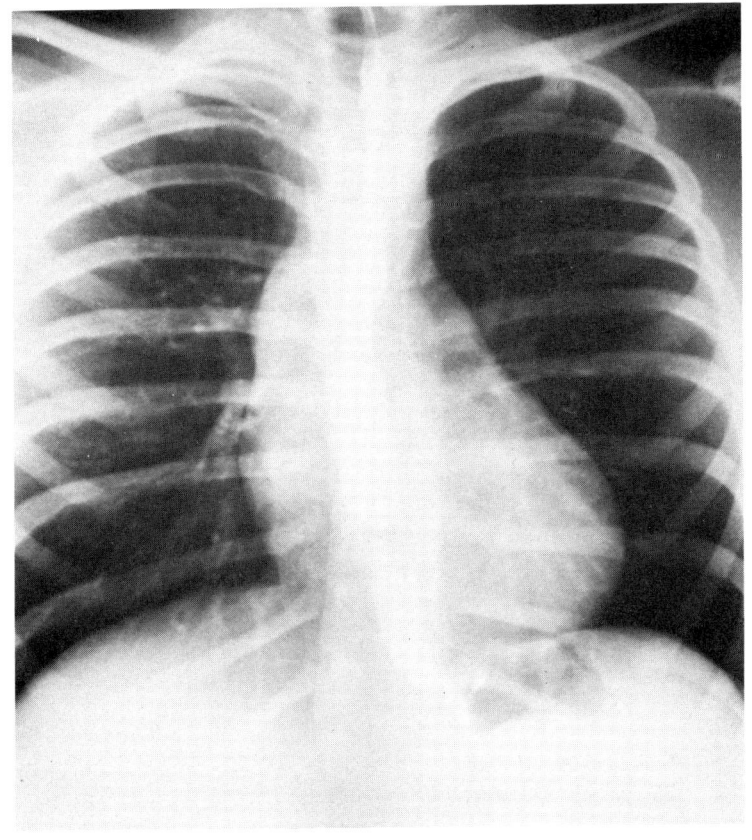

Figure 4.1

318. Figure 4.1 is the x-ray of an 8-year-old male who had easy fatigability and a soft, continuous murmur in the upper back. Electrocardiogram revealed minimal left ventricular hypertrophy. What is your diagnosis?
    A. Aortic stenosis
    B. Persistent ductus arteriosus
    C. Coarctation of the aorta
    D. Pulmonary valvar stenosis
    E. Peripheral pulmonary stenosis

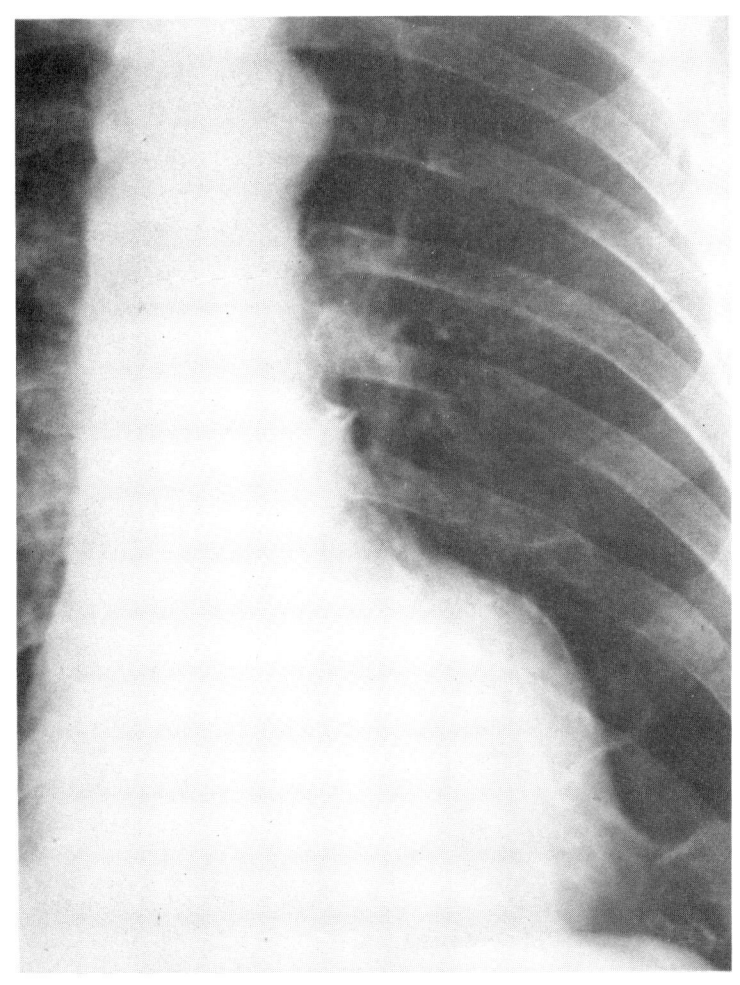

Figure 4.2

319. Figure 4.2 is an x-ray of an asymptomatic 48-year-old male executive coming in for his regular annual medical checkup. What is your diagnosis?
A. Calcific pericarditis
B. Left ventricular aneurysm
C. Hydatid cyst
D. Pleuropericarditis
E. Normal

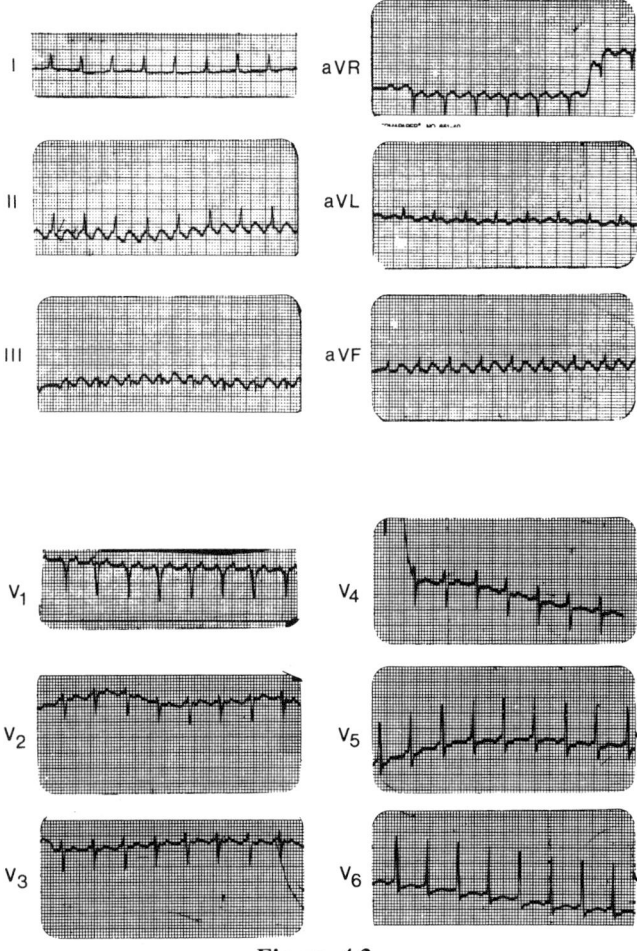

Figure 4.3

320. A 70-year-old man has dyspnea, orthopnea, and paroxysmal noctural dyspnea. He has generalized cardiomegaly and pulmonary and systemic venous hypertension. The EKG is shown in Figure 4.3. What is the cardiac rhythm?
   A. Ectopic atrial tachycardia
   B. Atrial flutter with 2:1 AV conduction
   C. Sinus tachycardia
   D. Supraventricular tachycardia
   E. Atrial fibrillation with rapid ventricular response

Diseases of the Cardiovascular System / 105

Figure 4.4

321. What is the rhythm in this lead tracing (Fig. 4.4)?
   A. First-degree heart block
   B. Second-degree heart block
   C. Third-degree heart block
   D. Ventricular premature beats
   E. Atrial premature beats

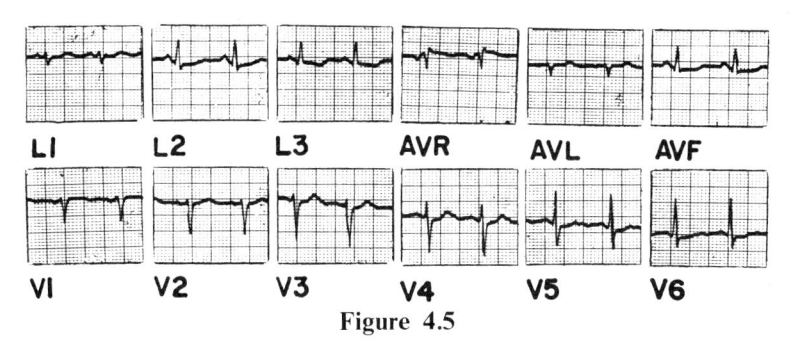

Figure 4.5

322. The patient is a 42-year-old woman with a history of many years of anterior chest pain of a somewhat atypical nature. The patient's pain has been present and relatively stable for a number of years, and the electrocardiographic picture shown in Figure 4.5 is a stable one. What is the diagnosis?
   A. Inferior wall infarction
   B. Anterior wall infarction
   C. Ventricular aneurysm
   D. Nonspecific changes
   E. Pericarditis

106 / Diseases of the Cardiovascular System

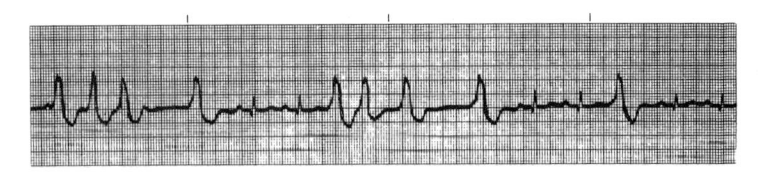

Figure 4.6

323. The electrocardiogram shown in Figure 4.6 was obtained during the initial stages of an acute myocardial infarction. What is the rhythm?
    A. Atrial fibrillation
    B. Atrial flutter
    C. Second-degree heart block
    D. Wenckebach phenomenon
    E. Ventricular tachycardia

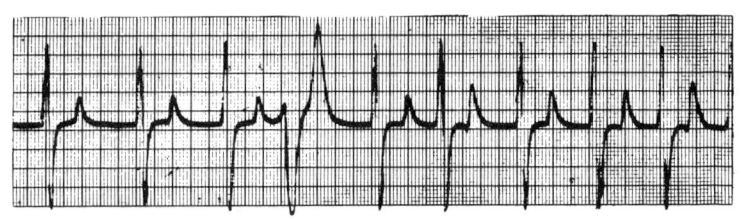

Figure 4.7

324. A 78-year-old man with advanced renal disease has the electrocardiogram shown in Figure 4.7 (lead II). What is the diagnosis?
    A. Hyperkalemia
    B. Hypercalcemia
    C. Hypernatremia
    D. Pericarditis
    E. Ventricular aneurysm

4. Diseases of the Cardiovascular System Answers and Comments

224. D. Wenckebach's AV block involves progressive P-Q lengthening and R-R shortening with dropped beat and repeat of the cycle. **(REF. 10, p. 546)**

225. D. The QRS complex may be insignificantly prolonged and the S-T segment and Q-T intervals shortened in hypercalcemia. **(REF. 10, p. 1560)**

226. D. The ventricular standby pacemaker functions when the heart rate falls below a present interval. If a QRS is not detected the pacemaker fires at a fixed rate until the inherent rhythm recovers. **(REF. 10, p. 1758)**

227. D. Occasionally there is right deviation of the electrical axis but never left deviation during an acute episode. **(REF. 10, p. 1036)**

228. C. Aortic stenosis is most likely to be associated with angina pectoris and syncope. Increased oxygen requirement, myocardial hypertrophy, low diastolic aortic pressure, and shortening of diastole are contributory factors to the syncope. **(REF. 10, p. 867)**

229. C. Peripheral neuropathy is not a complication of bacterial endocarditis. Many of the complications are thought to be embolic but may include vasculitis. **(REF. 10, p. 1256)**

230. D. The third heart sound is composed of weak vibrations of low frequency heard normally only in children and young adults. It is not heard in mitral stenosis. **(REF. 10, p. 229)**

231. D. Pericarditis secondary to transmural infarction has at least a 15% incidence and most cases appear within four days. **(REF. 10, p. 1127)**

232. A. Positively inotropic is the best description of the effect of calcium ions on the myocardium. Calcium plays a role in excitation-contraction coupling and in possible drug effects and in heart failure. (**REF.** 10, p. 68)

233. B. Pericardial effusion is a manifestation of myxedematous heart disease. Advanced myxedema is commonly associated with roentgenologic abnormalities and electrocardiographic changes. (**REF.** 10, p. 1385)

234. C. The temporary pacemaker is contraindicated in acute MI with pericardial rub and tachycardia. It should be recalled that there is a significant incidence of ventricular tachycardia with insertion of pacemakers. (**REF.** 10, p. 1757)

235. D. Pulmonary hypertension is associated with an increased density of the second heart sound which coincides with the end of the T wave on EKG. (**REF.** 10, p. 1225)

236. C. Sympathetic stimulation to the heart is mediated by release of norepinephrine. Parasympathetic innervation determines heart rate via acetylcholine release, and all impulses pass through the cardiac plexus. (**REF.** 10, p. 30)

237. D. The patient most likely has paroxysmal atrial tachycardia. Sinus tachycardia differs from atrial tachycardia in that it does not start or stop abruptly. (**REF.** 10, p. 497)

238. E. Significant Q waves are not a finding in myocarditis. In addition to the findings listed, sinus bradycardia, extrasystoles, atrial fibrillation, and flutter also occur in myocarditis. (**REF.** 10, p. 1286)

239. D. In the absence of coronary artery disease, angina pectoris occurs most frequently with aortic stenosis. Acute myocardial infarction is usually due to associated atherosclerotic coronary occlusion. (**REF.** 10, p. 867)

240. B. In aortic stenosis the first sound is usually normal but may be faint and of low pitch; the second is characteristically diminished. (**REF.** 10, p. 867)

241. B. Atrioventricular dissociation is independent beating of atria and ventricles and is recognized on electrocardiogram by fixed P-P and R-R intervals but variable P-R intervals. **(REF.** 10, p. 548)

242. A. Large a waves make one suspect that the right atrium is contracting against an increased resistance in the tricuspid valve or to right ventricular filling. Large a waves are not associated with patent ductus arteriosus. **(REF.** 10, p. 193)

243. C. Reversed splitting is not associated with prolongation of right ventricular systole. Delayed aortic closure allows P_2 to precede A_2; splitting is then maximal in expiration. **(REF.** 10, p. 219)

244. A. Of those listed, ventricular septal defect is most commonly involved with SBE, but patent ductus arteriosus may be more frequently involved. Less than 10% of cases of SBE are in congenitals. **(REF.** 10, p. 673)

245. B. An atrial flutter with 2:1 block most likely demonstrates an atrial rate of 300/min. The ventricular rates most commonly vary from 150 to 100. **(REF.** 10, p. 498)

246. E. One-third of patients "cured" died of heart failure in one series. **(REF.** 10, p. 1260)

247. A. The usual "window" theory fails to account for the fact that the abnormality is manifest before depolarization reaches the free wall of the left ventricle. **(REF.** 10, p. 260)

248. A. The myxoma is a solitary globular or polypoid tumor varying in size from that of a cherry to a peach. **(REF.** 10, p. 1403)

249. C. Exercise electrocardiography represents an increasingly popular noninvasive method for early detection of latent ischemic heart disease. **(REF.** 10, p. 335)

250. E. In rheumatic heart disease the mitral and aortic valves are the most commonly involved. Tricuspid disease is occasional and pulmonary valve disease is rare. **(REF.** 10, p. 857)

251. D. Small currents due to improper grounding may easily pass into the heart via an electrode catheter. All equipment should be grounded. **(REF.** 10, p. 365)

252. E. Scarlet fever does not generally cause late cardiac disease. Pericarditis in clinical practice is commonly idiopathic and frequently assumed to be of possible viral origin. **(REF.** 10, p. 1379)

253. D. Dye would show rapidly appearing in the left atrium, left ventricle, and the aorta. With cineangiography, the regurgitant jet is clearly visualized **(REF.** 10, p. 1861)

254. C. Left heart catheterization is a more accurate measurement but involves a slightly increased risk. **(REF.** 10, p. 1843)

255. A. Pulmonary blood flow is greater because of increased blood flow from the right atrium which receives blood from the vena cava and left atrium. **(REF.** 10, p. 659)

256. B. Echocardiography is not useful in the diagnosis of coarctation of the aorta. In addition to the conditions listed, this technique also detects ventricular hypertrophy, pericardial effusion, and atrial myxomas. **(REF.** 10, p. 318)

257. D. This pulse is seen in aortic regurgitation. The pressure in diastole is usually 50 mm Hg or lower. **(REF.** 10, p. 191)

258. E. Failure of the left ventricle most commonly causes failure of the right ventricle. The association is through pulmonary congestion and pulmonary hypertension. **(REF.** 10, p. 396)

259. E. Nausea and vomiting are not associated with mitral stenosis. The positive symptoms are associated with isolated left atrial and pulmonary venocapillary hypertension. **(REF.** 10, p. 892)

Diseases of the Cardiovascular System / 111

260. A. The most dramatic effects of digitalis are seen with congestive heart failure and atrial fibrillation. Digitalis is contraindicated in acute MI. **(REF.** 10, p. 429)

261. B. Atrioventricular dissociation and paroxysmal atrial tachycardia with block are distinctive manifestations of digitalis toxicity. **(REF.** 10, p. 434)

262. A. Chronic constrictive pericarditis is not found in association with rheumatic fever, although isolated cases have been reported with rheumatoid arthritis. **(REF.** 10, p. 1389)

263. E. Digitalis given in atrial flutter frequently causes atrial fibrillation, and quinidine given in atrial fibrillation may induce atrial flutter. **(REF.** 10, p. 567)

264. D. A regular tachycardia is not an atrial fibrillation. Sinus tachycardia differs from paroxysmal tachycardia in that it doesn't start or stop suddenly. **(REF.** 10, p. 497)

265. D. Retention of fluid is complex and not due to any one factor; however, hormones may contribute. Growth hormone does not have fluid-retaining properties. **(REF.** 10, p. 384)

266. H. Paroxysmal atrial tachycardia is a common form of recurrent palpitation associated with a rapid regular beat and an atrial rate of 140 to 220 per minute. **(REF.** 10, p. 526)

267. E. In atrial flutter with 2:1 block the atrial rate is about 300 per minute, and the block can be increased by vagotonic maneuvers. **(REF.** 10, p. 498)

268. F. In atrial fibrillation, the left atrial thrombi and systemic arterial emboli are increased in frequency, and the atrial rate is over 400 per minute. **(REF.** 10, p. 1488)

269. D. Ventricular flutter differs from ventricular tachycardia by the absence of distinct QRS and T waves. The ventricular flutter rate is 250 per minute. **(REF.** 10, p. 537)

270. G. In complete heart block there is virtual regularity of atrial and ventricular activity with variation of the P-R interval and a ventricular rate below 40 per minute. (**REF.** 10, p. 511)

271. A. Mitral stenosis is due to enlargement and hypertrophy of the left atrium and asynchronous atrial activation. (**REF.** 10, p. 897)

272. B. A prolonged P-R interval is the most frequent significant electrocardiographic abnormality in rheumatic fever. (**REF.** 10, p. 857)

273. E. In Wolff-Parkinson-White syndrome the P-R interval is short, the QRS is widened, and there is slurring of the upstroke of the R wave. (**REF.** 10, p. 532)

274. D. In hyperparathyroidism hypercalcemia may prolong the QRS and shorten the S-T and QT intervals. (**REF.** 10, p. 270)

275. C. In pericardial effusion there are low-voltage QRS complexes; T wave changes and persistent S-T elevation may also occur. (**REF.** 10, p. 1374)

276. C. The pain of myocardial infarction is usually described as a heaviness, tightness, or weight on the chest. The pain of pericarditis may be similar or of a sharper nature, but will occasionally be mild. (**REF.** 1, pp. 249, 300)

277. A. This scratchy sound is heard over the anterior precordium of most patients with acute pericarditis, but is found in less than 10% of patients with transmural myocardial infarction. (**REF.** 1, pp. 249, 303)

278. C. In acute myocardial infarction, prominent-peaked T-waves are followed by acute ST segment elevation and the development of significant Q waves. In pericarditis, ST segment elevation is unaccompanied by QRS complex changes. (**REF.** 1, pp. 249, 303)

279. C. In pericarditis, virtually all patients have inflammatory involvement of the subepicardial portion of the myocardium, accounting for the moderate enzyme elevations often seen. Enzyme elevations are characteristic of myocardial infarction. **(REF. 1, p. 303)**

280. A. Propranolol is well absorbed in the GI tract but undergoes extensive metabolism on its first pass through the liver, so that only 20% to 50% of the dose is bioavailable. Verapamil has very poor bioavailability and is used almost solely by intravenous route. **(REF. 1, p. 286)**

281. C. Both can result in severe hypotension, left ventricular failure, and cardiogenic shock in patients with left ventricular dysfunction. **(REF. 1, p. 286)**

282. B. Verapamil exerts a potent effect on the region of the sinus node and AV node, so that intravenous verapamil is highly effective in junctional tachycardias. **(REF. 1, p. 286)**

283. B. Verapamil appears to mediate its effect by interfering with movement of calcium through the so-called slow channel. **(REF. 1, p. 286)**

284. A. In the case of a single dropped P wave, the interval encompassing the dropped P wave is twice the basic sinus interval. **(REF. 1, pp. 278, 279)**

285. B. In this description of type I or Wenckebach second-degree heart block, the QRS is typically normal. **(REF. 1, p. 280)**

286. B. In the type II or Mobitz second-degree heart block, the P-P interval is regular and progression to complete heart block is common. **(REF. 1, p. 280)**

287. D. Digitalis may be a cause of both syndromes and is not indicated in their therapy. Pacemakers are inserted if bradycardia leads to heart failure. **(REF. 1, pp. 278, 280)**

288. B. Small R_1, deep S_2 and S_3 as well as inversion of T waves in at least three precordial leads may be seen. An operation may be indicated when there is a clearly expansile aneurysm. **(REF. 10, p. 327)**

289. C. In addition to dilatation of the proximal ascending aorta and normal overall cardiac size, there is also blunt rounding of the lower left cardiac contour in aortic stenosis. **(REF. 10, p. 279)**

290. A. A pulsative liver is not caused by aortic stenosis. For the other three conditions listed, simultaneous palpation of liver and carotid artery rules out transmitted pulsation. **(REF. 10, pp. 879, 292)**

291. B. Coarctation of the aorta and aortic occlusive disease may cause blood pressure in the arms to differ from pressure in the legs. Improper cuff size, dissection of the aorta, abdominal aneurysm, and infants under 1 year of age are other conditions affecting the BP difference. **(REF. 10, p. 709)**

292. B. EKG signs include left axis deviation and high voltage of the QRS complex in V_5 and V_6, as well as deep S in V_1 and V_2 and prolonged QRS in the left precordial leads. **(REF 10, p. 269)**

293. C. High urinary specific gravity, albuminuria, nocturia, and oliguria occur in untreated, uncomplicated congestive heart failure. **(REF. 10, p. 411)**

294. A. In addition to the first three signs listed, low voltage as manifested by diminished QRS size may also occur. **(REF. 10, p. 1374)**

295. D. Paroxysmal atrial fibrillation may be found secondary to hyperthyroid heart disease. Thyroid may affect the heart muscle directly or there may be excessive sympathetic stimulation. **(REF. 10, pp. 1549–1550)**

296. A. Digitalis slows the ventricular rate by a depressant

Diseases of the Cardiovascular System / 115

action on the ventricular myocardial tissue. Diminishing of frequency of impulses bombarding the ventricles is the result. (**REF.** 10, p. 426)

297. A. Careful monitoring is essential for reduced morbidity. In addition to the first three listed, other end points include S-T segment changes, multiple premature beats, drop in blood pressure, and cerebral hypoxia. (**REF.** 10, p. 359)

298. B. The ventricular rate will be regular if there is complete heart block or ventricular tachycardia. In the latter, the ventricle responds to a regular ectopic rhythm. (**REF.** 10, p. 499)

299. A. Type II hyperlipoproteinemia may be secondary to the first three conditions listed. A high risk of atherosclerosis is associated with this pattern. (**REF.** 10, p. 956)

300. B. The symptomatology depends on the quantity of effusion and the rate of development of the effusion. The diagnostic triad for pericardial effusion is rising venous pressure, falling arterial pressure, and a small quiet heart. (**REF.** 10, p. 1373)

301. E. Diagnostic evaluation should include all four listings. Essential hypertension is commonly associated with a strong family history, but absence does not rule it out. (**REF.** 10, p. 1175)

302. A. The symptoms and signs are like any sudden paroxysmal tachycardia, but the ventricular rate is the clue, after carotid pressure, to the diagnosis of atrial flutter with 2:1 block. (**REF.** 10, pp. 498–499)

303. E. The maneuvers listed increase the block and are useful for diagnosis, not for converting the atrial flutter to a sinus rhythm. (**REF.** 10, pp. 498–499)

304. A. Digitalis slows the ventricular rate and controls or prevents heart failure. (**REF.** 10, pp. 498–499)

305. C. The tachycardia is not commonly associated with syphilitic heart disease. The sudden change to half rate on vagal stimulation is diagnostic of atrial flutter with 2:1 block. **(REF.** 10, pp. 498-499)

306. E. All of the first four complications are common in arrhythmia, but pericarditis is not seen. The attacks of flutter are often more complicated than atrial tachycardia because of their tendency to persist. **(REF.** 10, pp. 498-499)

307. B. Pericarditis with effusion is the most likely diagnosis. The normal pericardial sac contains 50 cc of fluid, and maximal capacity without damage is 100 to 150 cc. **(REF.** 10, pp. 1372-1378)

308. E. Hyperthyroidism is not associated with pericarditis with effusion. Association of pericarditis with myocardial infarction may be more common than suspected, but pericarditis as detected clinically is usually idiopathic. **(REF.** 10, pp. 1372-1378)

309. A. Physical signs do not include giant a waves in the neck. The cervical veins are engorged and may pulsate, but the head of the fluid column is often hidden. **(REF.** 10, pp. 1372-1378)

310. B. Elevation of the S-T segment in the standard leads is the most consistent and significant alteration. T wave changes also occur, and there may be diminution of QRS complex. **(REF.** 10, p. 1374)

311. D. Pericardiocentesis is the best treatment. Cardiac tamponade is the indication for pericardial tap, usually associated with delay in diagnosis or treatment. **(REF.** 10, pp. 1372-1378)

312. C. Pericarditis is the most likely diagnosis. The pain may be sternal or parasternal, and radiate to posterior or anterior cervical areas, to either trapezius, or to either shoulder. **(REF.** 10, pp. 1372-1378)

313. D. Viruses include Coxsackie B, ECHO 8, mumps, and infectious mononucleosis. (**REF.** 10, pp. 1372–1378)

314. C. The events of the third day were probably caused by cardiac tamponade. The diagnosis of tuberculosis must always be considered. (**REF.** 10, pp. 1372–1378)

315. B. Pericardiocentesis would be the correct treatment. Open pericardial biopsy is performed if there is uncertainty as to diagnosis or there is no response to therapy. (**REF.** 10, pp. 1372–1378)

316. C. A water-bottle heart would probably be revealed. The association of clear lung fields with a large cardiac silhouette distinguishes pericardial effusion from heart failure. (**REF.** 10, pp. 1372–1378)

317. C. Essential hypertension is the most likely diagnosis. A secondary cause for hypertension is found in only 10% of patients, with 90% labeled as "essential." (**REF.** 10, p. 1175)

318. C. Coarctation of the aorta is the diagnosis. There is a "reverse 3" deformity of the esophagus, the belly of which represents the dilated aorta after the coarctation. The border of the descending aorta shows a medial indentation called the "3" or "tuck" sign, the belly of the "3" representing the poststenotic dilation and the upper portion by the dilated subclavian artery and small transverse aortic arch. (**REF.** 10, p. 709)

319. B. Note the abnormal humped contour of the left ventricular border, with a curvilinear calcification following the abnormal cardiac contour. The presence of calcification in the ventricular wall and the abnormal left ventricular contour alert one to the consideration of a ventricular aneurysm. (**REF.** 10, p. 1706)

320. B. The cardiac rhythm is atrial flutter with 2:1 AV conduction. QRS complexes occur with perfect regularity at a rate of about 150/min. Their normal contour and duration in-

118 / Diseases of the Cardiovascular System

dicate that ventricular activation occurs normally via the AV junction-His-Purkinje system. **(REF.** 10, p. 528)

321. B. The P-R interval of the first two complexes is normal at 0.20 sec. The QRS duration is 0.16 sec. The third P wave is nonconducted. This cycle recurs in the remainder of the strip. This is second-degree heart block of the Mobitz type II variety. Note the wide QRS. When this type of heart block develops, either de novo or in the course of an acute myocardial infarction, a cardiac pacemaker is usually recommended, as the incidence of complete heart block is high in this situation. **(REF.** 10, p. 544)

322. D. The S-T is depressed in leads II, III, AVF, and V_{4-6}. These nonspecific abnormalities do not indicate significant coronary heart disease, especially in an apprehensive young patient. **(REF.** 10, p. 1029)

323. E. The rhythm is regular sinus rhythm with a rate of 85 beats/min. The sinus rhythm is interrupted frequently by bursts of irregular ventricular, premature beats. Sinus rhythm is uninterrupted as can be determined by plotting the P-P intervals which are regular. The rhythm may be termed a chaotic ventricular arrhythmia or ventricular tachycardia. Its gross irregularity is unusual. Antiarrhythmic therapy is indicated. **(REF.** 10, p. 508)

324. A. No atrial activity is detected. The ventricular rate is slightly irregular. Beat no. 4 is a ventricular premature contraction. The T waves are tall and markedly peaked. This type of T wave is characteristic of hyperkalemia as is absence of visible atrial activity. The potassium level was 8.2 mg%. **(REF.** 10, p. 1600)

5. Diseases of the Blood

DIRECTIONS: Each of the questions or incomplete statements below is followed by five suggested answers or completions. Select the **one** that is **best** in each case.

325. A patient with chronic myelogenous leukemia who develops left upper quadrant pain radiating to the left shoulder probably has
    A. splenic infarction
    B. perforated gastric ulcer
    C. pancreatitis
    D. ischemic colitis
    E. renal stone

326. Cryoglobulinemia may be found in association with all of the following EXCEPT
    A. multiple myeloma
    B. lymphosarcoma
    C. systemic lupus
    D. infectious mononucleosis
    E. thalassemia

327. Acute myeloblastic leukemia (AML) is characterized by
    A. peak incidence in childhood
    B. high leukocyte alkaline phosphatase
    C. Philadelphia chromosome
    D. Auer bodies in blast cells
    E. response to vincristine and prednisone

120 / Diseases of the Blood

328. All of the following are generally associated with secondary polycythemia EXCEPT
   A. Cushing's syndrome
   B. uterine myomata
   C. hypernephroma
   D. gastric malignancy
   E. cerebellar hemangiomas

329. All of the following hemoglobins migrate slower on paper electrophoresis than type A hemoglobin EXCEPT
   A. S
   B. C
   C. D
   D. Barts
   E. A_2

330. Infectious mononucleosis is characterized by all of the following EXCEPT
   A. antibodies to EB virus
   B. heterophil antibodies
   C. antinuclear antibodies
   D. anti-I antibodies
   E. antibodies to sheep red cells

331. Normal hemoglobin molecules are composed of
   A. two alpha and two beta chains
   B. one alpha and one beta chain
   C. four alpha chains
   D. four beta chains
   E. two alpha and two delta chains

332. All of the following purpuras have thrombocytopenia EXCEPT
   A. idiopathic thrombocytopenia purpura
   B. disseminated lupus erythematosus
   C. infectious purpura (e.g., rubeola, varicella)
   D. acute leukemia
   E. Henoch-Schönlein purpura

Diseases of the Blood / 121

333. Hemophilia A can be characterized by
    A. normal immunoreactive Factor VIII
    B. normal functional Factor VIII
    C. decreased immunoreactive Factor VIII
    D. prolonged bleeding time
    E. platelet function abnormality

334. Patients homozygous for hemoglobin C may manifest all of the following EXCEPT
    A. increased target cells
    B. increased spleen size
    C. intracellular crystals
    D. increased osmotic fragility
    E. marrow hyperplasia

335. Multiple myeloma is often associated with all of the following EXCEPT
    A. bone pain
    B. osteoblastic bone lesions
    C. Bence Jones proteinuria
    D. occurrence after age forty in most cases
    E. myeloma cells in bone marrow

336. The intracellular inclusions in hemoglobin H disease are due to precipitated
    A. alpha chains
    B. beta chains
    C. gamma chains
    D. delta chains
    E. epsilon chains

337. Thrombocythemia can be distinguished from reactive thrombocytosis by
    A. increased megakaryocyte number
    B. increased total platelet mass
    C. increased platelet turnover
    D. normal platelet survival
    E. thromboembolism and hemorrhage

338. Eosinophilia is frequently seen with all of the following EXCEPT
    A. allergic disorders
    B. parasitic infestations
    C. Löffler's syndrome
    D. following irradiation
    E. ACTH administration

339. Multiple myeloma is commonly associated with all of the following EXCEPT
    A. elevated serum calcium
    B. anemia
    C. elevated serum alkaline phosphatase
    D. elevated erythrocyte sedimentation rate
    E. elevated serum globulin

340. Sickle cell anemia is usually associated with all of the following EXCEPT
    A. hemoglobin S
    B. small or normal-sized spleen
    C. normal reticulocyte count
    D. shortened erythrocyte life span
    E. normal hemoglobin concentration in the red blood cell

341. Patients with coagulation abnormality due to liver disease are likely to have
    A. thrombocytosis
    B. prolonged bleeding time
    C. short partial thromboplastin time
    D. prolonged prothrombin time
    E. deficiency of Factor VIII

342. A man with a prosthetic aortic valve is most likely to have hemolysis from
    A. thermal injury
    B. isoantibodies
    C. autoantibodies
    D. red cell fragmentation
    E. hemoglobinopathy

Diseases of the Blood / 123

343. An Italian boy with splenomegaly and a microcytic anemia showing target cells will also have
    A. normal hemoglobin electrophoresis
    B. an MCV greater than 90
    C. cortical thinning of long bones
    D. sickle cell crises
    E. iron deficiency

344. Iron deficiency in infancy may be due to all of the following except
    A. low birth weight
    B. hemolysis
    C. early clamping of cord
    D. inadequate diet
    E. blood loss

345. Chronic myelocytic leukemia has all of the following characteristics EXCEPT
    A. slight to moderate lymph node enlargement
    B. marked splenomegaly
    C. frequent complication of herpes zoster
    D. sternal tenderness
    E. palpable liver

346. The presence of increased levels of 2,3-DPG in the red cell is associated with
    A. hemolytic anemia due to sulfa drugs
    B. increased oxygen affinity
    C. decreased oxygen affinity
    D. loss of red cell energy
    E. multiple congenital abnormalities

124 / Diseases of the Blood

347. All of the following statements are true EXCEPT
  A. people with group AB red blood cells have anti-A and anti-B sera
  B. group O, Rh negative red blood cells are "universal donors"
  C. the red blood cells of 85% of Caucasians are agglutinated by anti-Rh serum
  D. the genotype for group B red blood cells may be BB or BO
  E. the genotype for group O red blood cells is only OO

348. Helmet cells and other schistocytes are suggestive of
  A. microangiopathic hemolytic anemia
  B. thalassemia
  C. megaloblastic anemia
  D. iron deficiency anemia
  E. schistosomiasis

349. Hemolytic anemias are usually associated with all of the following EXCEPT
  A. erythroid hypoplasia of the marrow
  B. decreased red cell survival
  C. increased numbers of reticulocytes
  D. increased fecal urobilinogen
  E. increased urine urobilinogen

350. All of the following statements are true of methemoglobin EXCEPT
  A. it does not combine with oxygen
  B. it may be produced by such toxic agents as nitrites, sulfonamides, aniline, phenacetin, or nitrates which become converted to nitrites
  C. cyanosis, headaches, vertigo, mental confusion, and a desire to sleep may result from usage
  D. it may be changed to normal hemoglobin by methylene blue
  E. it contains a ferrous porphyrin complex

351. Hypochromic microcytic anemia is seen in all of the following EXCEPT
    A. chronic blood loss
    B. thalassemia
    C. thiamine deficiency
    D. pyridoxine deficiency
    E. iron deficiency

352. All of the following are findings of lead intoxication EXCEPT
    A. increased urinary excretion of coproporphyrin III
    B. Howell-Jolly bodies
    C. basophilic stippling
    D. bone marrow aplasia
    E. "lead line" on the gingiva

353. Elevated platelet counts may be found in all of the following EXCEPT
    A. splenectomized patients
    B. acute hemorrhage
    C. the postoperative period
    D. chronic granulocytic leukemia
    E. penicillin allergy

354. The synthesis of heme requires all of the following EXCEPT
    A. glycine
    B. urate
    C. iron
    D. protoporphyrin
    E. mitochondria

126 / Diseases of the Blood

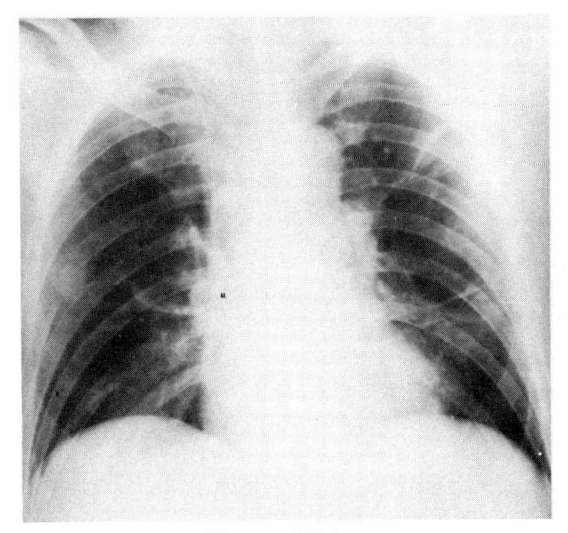

Figure 5.1,A

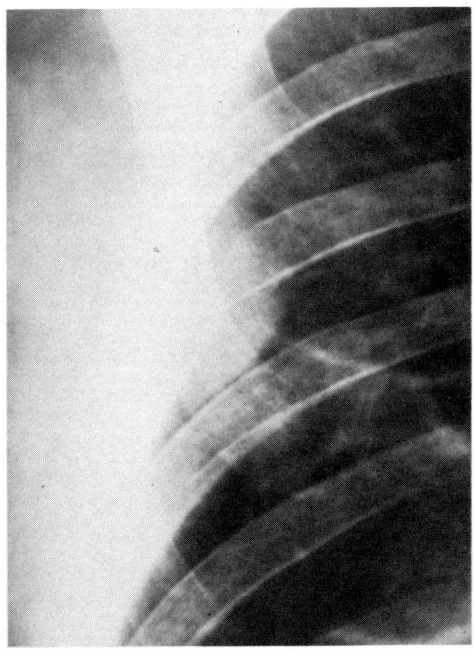

Figure 5.1,B

Diseases of the Blood / 127

355. Figures 5.1, A and B, are the x-rays of a 60-year-old white male with pain in the right chest. What is your diagnosis?
    A. Aneurysmal bone cyst
    B. Multiple myeloma
    C. Lymphosarcoma
    D. Prostatic metastases
    E. Hyperparathyroidism

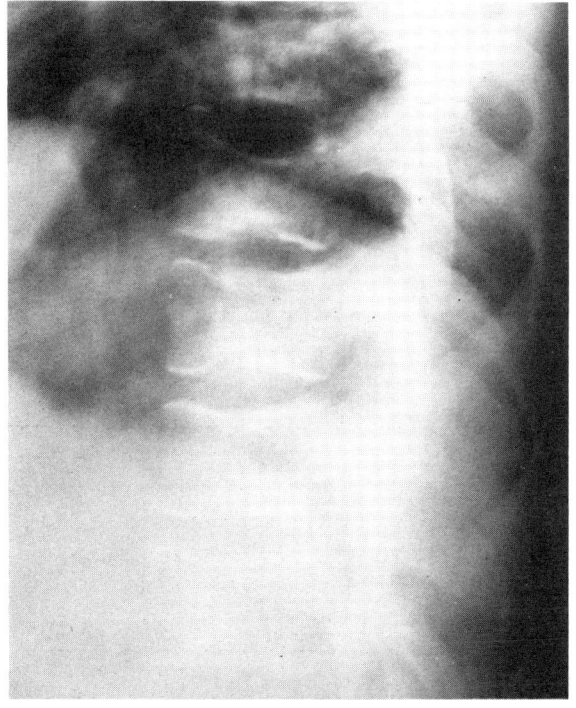

Figure 5.2

356. Figure 5.2 is the x-ray of a 30-year-old black female with recurrent abdominal pain and pallor. What is your diagnosis?
    A. Sickle cell anemia
    B. Hemangioma
    C. Spondylitis deformans
    D. Ankylosing spondylitis
    E. Multiple myeloma

128 / Diseases of the Blood

Case Work-up

Blood film	Polychromatophilia, some spherocytes
Bilirubin	2.0 mg/100 ml total 0.3 mg/100 ml direct
Haptoglobin	10 mg/100 ml
Lactate dehydrogenase	200 IU/liter
Urine bilirubin	Negative
Antiglobulin test	Positive direct Negative indirect

357. The case work-up shown above is of a 30-year-old woman presenting with a hemoglobin of 6.0 gm/100 ml. The most likely diagnosis is
   A. iron deficiency
   B. congenital spherocytosis
   C. liver failure and hemolysis
   D. splenomegaly and hemolysis
   E. autoimmune hemolytic anemia

DIRECTIONS: Each group of questions below consists of a list of lettered headings followed by a list of numbered words, phrases or statements. For **each** numbered word, phrase or statement, select the **one** lettered heading that is most closely associated with it. Each lettered heading may be selected once, more than once, or not at all.

   A. Beta thalassemia major
   B. Hemoglobin H disease
   C. Sickle cell disease
   D. Hemoglobin C disease
   E. Hemoglobin M disease

358. Forms tactoids or liquid crystals when hypoxic

Diseases of the Blood / 129

359. A mild hemolytic anemia with intraerythrocytic crystals seen on fixed blood smears

360. May result from defect in processing of globin messenger RNA

361. Decreased alpha chain production leads to four-beta tetramer formation

362. Bone infarction can occur that may be difficult to distinguish from osteomyelitis

---

DIRECTIONS: Each set of lettered headings below is followed by a list of numbered words or phrases. For each numbered word or phrase select
    A if the item is associated with (A) *only,*
    B if the item is associated with (B) *only,*
    C if the item is associated with *both* (A) *and* (B),
    D if the item is associated with *neither* (A) *nor* (B).

    A. Primary polycythemia
    B. Chronic myelogenous leukemia
    C. Both
    D. Neither

363. Elevated levels of serum vitamin B_{12}

364. Probably a clonal disease originating from a single multipotential stem cell

365. Frequently presents with a low platelet count

366. Myelofibrosis is often seen in the late stages

130 / Diseases of the Blood

DIRECTIONS: For each of the questions or incomplete statements below, **one** or **more** of the answers or completions given is correct. Select

- A if only *1, 2 and 3* are correct,
- B if only *1 and 3* are correct,
- C if only *2 and 4* are correct,
- D if only *4* is correct,
- E if *all* are correct.

367. Patients with malignant lymphoma receiving long-term therapy with vincristine may develop
    1. loss of the achilles tendon reflex
    2. muscle pains
    3. paresthesias
    4. diplopia

368. Hemoglobin S is characterized by
    1. alpha chain substitution
    2. intracellular crystallization
    3. fast migration at pH 8.6
    4. hydrophobic bonding in the reduced state

369. The sickle cell trait may include
    1. vascular occlusive phenomena under stress
    2. renal concentration defect
    3. positive sickle preparation
    4. hematuria

370. In the macrocytic anemia of pregnancy
    1. it occurs most commonly in the third trimester of pregnancy
    2. it responds to folic acid
    3. the anemia disappears spontaneously on interruption or termination of pregnancy
    4. splenomegaly present in about one-third of cases

Diseases of the Blood / 131

371. Hemolytic disease of the newborn (erythroblastosis fetalis) due to Rh incompatibility is usually associated with
    1. a positive direct Coombs' test using the baby's red blood cells
    2. a positive direct Coombs' test using the mother's red blood cells
    3. a positive indirect Coombs' test using the mother's serum
    4. toxemia of pregnancy

372. Elevation of the serum iron-binding capacity may occur in association with
    1. iron deficiency
    2. late pregnancy
    3. acute hepatitis
    4. chronic infection

373. Decreased osmotic fragility is found in
    1. hereditary spherocytosis
    2. thalassemia minor
    3. acquired hemolytic anemia
    4. iron deficiency anemia

374. Hemolytic anemia due to intravascular red cell destruction may be associated with
    1. paroxysmal nocturnal hemoglobinuria
    2. ABO isoantibodies and transfusion
    3. clostridial sepsis
    4. glucose-6-phosphate dehydrogenase deficiency and drugs

375. Hereditary persistence of hemoglobin F can be characterized as
    1. cause of sickling of red cells
    2. disease of infants only
    3. variant of thalassemia major
    4. benign genetic abnormality

132 / Diseases of the Blood

Directions Summarized				
A	B	C	D	E
1,2,3 only	1,3 only	2,4 only	4 only	All are correct

376. Typical findings in the peripheral blood of patients with splenectomy include
    1. macrophages
    2. nucleated red cells and target cells
    3. leukopenia
    4. Howell-Jolly bodies

377. Although type O blood is considered to be the universal donor, there are certain dangers in this practice such as
    1. at times patients with type A_2 blood may be mistyped as type O
    2. type O donors have a higher incidence of serum hepatitis
    3. type O donors have high titers of anti-A and anti-B in their plasma
    4. type O cells have a shorter survival time when transfused than do other cell types

378. The anemia of thalassemia is due to
    1. decreased globin chain production
    2. production of an abnormal hemoglobin
    3. increased red cell destruction
    4. stem cell failure

379. Contact activation of the coagulation mechanism
    1. involves the intrinsic pathway
    2. depends on Factor VII
    3. depends on Factor XII
    4. is poor on glass surfaces

Diseases of the Blood / 133

DIRECTIONS: This section consists of situations, each followed by a series of questions. Study each situation, and select the **one** best answer to each question following it.

CASE 1 (Questions 380-384): A 50-year-old white female presents with a three-week history of tiredness and pallor. A family member has noted some yellowness of her eyes, but she denies darkening of the urine. Physical examination reveals only slight jaundice. Laboratory data include a Hb of 9 gm, reticulocyte count of 12%, a bilirubin in the serum of 2 mgm% indirect reacting, and some microspherocytes on peripheral smear.

380. The most likely cause of this woman's anemia is
 A. blood loss externally
 B. decreased red cell production
 C. ineffective erythropoiesis
 D. intravascular hemolysis
 E. extravascular hemolysis

381. Spherocytosis may be associated with all of the following EXCEPT
 A. burns
 B. hereditary spherocytosis
 C. Coombs'-positive hemolytic anemia
 D. glucose-6-phosphate dehydrogenase deficiency
 E. splenomegaly

382. All of the following may be expected in this case EXCEPT
 A. depressed haptoglobin level
 B. increased bilirubin in the urine
 C. increased urobilinogen in the stool
 D. increased methemalbumin in the blood
 E. decreased hemopexin in the blood

134 / Diseases of the Blood

383. Bone marrow examination is most likely to show
    A. megaloblastic changes
    B. giant metamyelocytes
    C. increased erythroid to myeloid ratio
    D. increased lymphocytes
    E. shift to left of the myeloid series

384. Other changes in a peripheral blood smear might include all of the following EXCEPT
    A. large polychromatophilic cells
    B. normoblasts
    C. leukocytosis
    D. basophilic stippling
    E. hypochromia

CASE 2 (Questions 385-389): A 57-year-old man with a history of chronic alcohol ingestion is admitted to the hospital with acute alcoholic intoxication and lobar pneumonia. Physical examination reveals pallor; a large, tender liver; and consolidation of the right lower lobe. Laboratory data include an Hb of 7 gm, WBC of 4000, and platelet count of 85,000.

385. Likely causes for anemia in this man include all of the following EXCEPT
    A. hemorrhagic diathesis
    B. gastrointestinal bleeding
    C. nutritional deficiency
    D. toxic marrow suppression
    E. hemoglobinopathy

386. The most likely vitamin deficiency related to the pancytopenia is
    A. B_{12}
    B. folate
    C. pyridoxine
    D. thiamine
    E. riboflavin

387. Toxic marrow suppression is most likely to affect
    A. developing erythrocytes and myelocytes
    B. mature polymorphonuclear leukocytes
    C. mature red cells
    D. mature platelets
    E. eosinophils

388. Examination of the peripheral smear might show all of the following EXCEPT
    A. target cells
    B. macrocytosis
    C. spur cells
    D. increased platelet adhesiveness
    E. increased segmentation of white cells

389. A deficiency of coagulation factors in this patient would most likely be due to Factors
    A. V and VIII
    B. VIII, IX, XI, XII
    C. XIII
    D. II, VII, X, V
    E. I, V, VIII

136 / Diseases of the Blood

CASE 3 (Questions 390-394): A 55-year-old man comes to you because of headaches, dizziness, lassitude, weakness, ringing in his ears, and several episodes of transitory dimness of his vision. The onset of these symptoms has been insidious during the past several months. He has also noted that his complexion has become quite ruddy and his eyes "bloodshot" for several months. Physical examination is unremarkable except for the following findings: the face appears somewhat reddened and the fingers and toes are almost cyanotic. The liver is 1 in. below the right costal margin. The spleen tip is palpable on deep inspiration. On examination of the fundi, the vessels are engorged and the retina is deeply colored. There is no abnormality of heart or lungs. Laboratory data reveal the following results: chest x-ray is normal; urinalysis is normal; hemoglobin is 20 gm%; hematocrit is 53%; red blood count is 7,500,000; white blood count is 16,500; platelet count is 800,000. A differential showed 55% segmented neutrophils, 10% bands, 4% metamyelocytes, 1% eosinophils, 1% basophils, 27% lymphocytes, and 2% monocytes. There are three nucleated red blood cells per 100 white blood cells. Erythrocyte sedimentation rate was 2 mm in one hour.

390. The most likely diagnosis is
  A. polycythemia vera
  B. stress erythrocytosis
  C. secondary polycythemia
  D. chronic myelocytic leukemia
  E. agnogenic myeloid metaplasia

391. Which of the following procedures would be most important to help prove the diagnosis?
  A. Splenic aspiration
  B. Bone marrow aspiration
  C. Bone marrow biopsy
  D. Schilling test
  E. Measurement of red cell mass and plasma volume

392. A good mode of therapy would most likely be
    A. phenobarbital
    B. radioactive phosphorus
    C. splenectomy
    D. oxygen therapy under positive pressure
    E. nitrogen mustard

393. Common complications of the disease include all of the following EXCEPT
    A. secondary gout
    B. visual disturbances
    C. duodenal ulcer
    D. hemolytic crisis
    E. vascular thrombosis

394. Which of the following is most important in distinguishing polycythemia vera from polycythemia seen secondary to chronic cor pulmonale?
    A. Normal arterial oxygen saturation
    B. Elevated leukocyte alkaline phosphatase
    C. Increased red cell mass
    D. Increased blood viscosity
    E. Red cell count over 7,000,000

CASE 4 (Questions 395-399): An 18-year-old male of Italian extraction is found to have a hypochromic microcytic anemia of 10 gm%. In addition there is a fair degree of anisocytosis, poikilocytosis, and targeting on smear. The white blood count is 9,500, the platelet count is 240,000, and the reticulocyte count is 7%. The spleen is palpated 5 cm below the left costal margin.

395. Which of the following is the most likely diagnosis?
    A. Sickle cell trait
    B. Thalassemia minor
    C. Hemoglobin S-C disease
    D. Iron deficiency anemia
    E. Hereditary spherocytosis

138 / Diseases of the Blood

396. Which of the following would be most helpful in distinguishing this case from one of pure iron deficiency anemia?
    A. Peripheral blood smear
    B. Osmotic fragility test
    C. Ham test
    D. Hemoglobin electrophoresis on paper
    E. Serum iron determination

397. One would expect to find which of the following in thalassemia minor?
    A. An increased amount of fetal or A_2 hemoglobin
    B. Increased osmotic fragility of the red cells
    C. Absent bone marrow iron
    D. Increased macroglobulins in the serum
    E. Small amounts of S hemoglobin

398. The present treatment of choice for thalassemia minor is
    A. splenectomy
    B. removal of the abnormal hemoglobin pigment
    C. purely supportive
    D. plasmapheresis
    E. intramuscular iron

399. Which of the following abnormal hemoglobins characteristically produces targeting in the peripheral blood?
    A. Hemoglobin M
    B. Hemoglobin S
    C. Hemoglobin Zurich
    D. Hemoglobin C
    E. Hemoglobin Barts

5. Diseases of the Blood
   Answers and Comments

325. A. The patient probably has splenic infarction. Rupture of the spleen may also occur and has been reported as the presenting sign. **(REF. 4, p. 1565)**

326. E. Cryoglobulinemia may be found in association with the first four conditions cited. An association with thalassemia would be unusual. Cryoglobulins are serum proteins that undergo reversible precipitation at low temperature. Hyperviscosity syndromes may result. **(REF. 4, p. 1788)**

327. D. Auer bodies are slender, pink, staining rods containing lysozyme and are exclusively seen in AML. **(REF. 4, p. 1536)**

328. D. Gastric malignancy is not associated with secondary polycythemia. The other tumors listed generally are thought to produce endogenous erythropoietin and are distinguished from primary polycythemia by high levels of erythropoietin. **(REF. 4, p. 991)**

329. D. Barts hemoglobin does not migrate slower than type A. Other fast hemoglobins include H, I, J, K, and N. **(REF. 4, p. 818)**

330. C. Antinuclear antibodies are not characteristic of infectious mononucleosis. Heterophil antibodies react against sheep red cells and are not absorbed out by guinea pig kidney. **(REF. 4, p. 1363)**

331. A. Normal hemoglobin molecules are composed of two alpha and two beta chains. The peptide chains are so arranged that the complete molecule is formed of a tetramer of two equal halves. **(REF. 4, p. 88)**

332. E. Henoch-Schonlein purpura does not have thrombocytopenia. The basic lesion in Henoch-Schonlein purpura is an inflammatory process involving mainly the capillaries and arterioles. **(REF. 4, p. 1074)**

333. A. Antibodies to Factor VIII detect normal quantities in hemophilia A, but function of the molecule is abnormal. **(REF. 4, p. 1160)**

334. D. Homozygous C red cells are often target-shaped with "extra" membrane to make them more resistant to osmotic fragility. **(REF. 4, p. 856)**

335. B. Bone lesions in myeloma are destructive, but the alkaline phosphatase is usually normal, indicating little blastic activity. **(REF. 4, p. 1739)**

336. B. Hemoglobin H is seen in alpha-thalassemia, in which decreased production of alpha chains leads to excess of beta chains. **(REF. 4, p. 877)**

337. E. Reactive thrombocytosis is usually transitory, without thromboembolism, hemorrhage, splenomegaly, or leukocytosis. **(REF. 4, p. 1129)**

338. E. Steroids cause decreased numbers of eosinophils to circulate, so that eosinophilia may be seen in Addison's disease, for example. **(REF. 4, p. 1298)**

339. C. Diffuse osteoporosis or discrete, punched-out lesions may occur, and the alkaline phosphatase does not rise. **(REF. 4, p. 1739)**

340. C. Since sickle cell anemia is a chronic hemolytic anemia, the reticulocyte is chronically elevated except in aplastic crises. **(REF. 4, p. 836)**

341. D. These patients are likely to have prolonged prothrombin time. Deficiencies of Factors V, X, prothrombin, and fibrinogen explain these results. **(REF. 4, p. 1210)**

342. D. Most valves associated with hemolysis have been aortic, but mitral prostheses or unsuccessful mitral valvuloplasty have caused red cell fragmentation. **(REF. 4, p. 960)**

343. C. Striking skeletal changes may be seen, including thickening of the skull and widening of long bones. **(REF. 4, p. 880)**

344. B. Iron deficiency in infancy is not due to hemolysis. Sixty percent of body iron concentration at birth is contained in circulating hemoglobin. **(REF. 4, p. 626)**

345. C. Herpes zoster infections are more common in diseases with loss of cell-mediated immunity such as Hodgkin's disease. **(REF. 4, p. 1792)**

346. C. 2, 3-DPG binds to the central cavity of the heme molecule and changes the configuration in favor of oxygen release. **(REF. 4, p. 1004)**

347. A. Group AB has neither anti-A nor anti-B, since both A and B antigens are on the red cells. **(REF. 4, p. 455)**

348. A. Schistocytes are suggestive of microangiopathic hemolytic anemia. Helmet cells and schistocytes are traumatic types of red cell damage such as are seen in malignant hypertension or disseminated intravascular fibrosis. **(REF. 4, p. 960)**

349. A. Hemolytic anemias are not associated with erythroid hypoplasia of the marrow. Erythroid hyperplasia is present except during infections or insults that lead to aregenerative crises. **(REF. 4, p. 747)**

350. E. Hemoglobin is converted to methemoglobin by oxidation of ferrous iron to its ferric state. **(REF. 4, p. 1011)**

351. C. Microcytic hypochromic anemias are caused by disorders of iron, globin, heme, or porphyrin metabolism and are not seen in thiamine deficiency. **(REF. 4, p. 624)**

142 / Diseases of the Blood

352. D. Bone marrow aplasia is not a finding of lead intoxication. Symptoms also include abdominal pain, constipation, vomiting, and muscle weakness. **(REF. 4, p. 662)**

353. E. Elevated platelet counts may be found in the first four conditions listed. Penicillin allergy may lower platelet counts. Reactive thrombocytosis is rarely associated with thromboembolic or hemorrhagic phenomena. **(REF. 4, p. 1129)**

354. B. Heme synthesis does not require urate. Mitochondria participate in the first and last steps of heme synthesis, with middle steps occurring in solution. **(REF. 4, p. 119)**

355. B. There is lytic destruction of the sixth rib with a pathologic fracture and an extrapleural mass. The most common manifestation of multiple myeloma is multiple, "punched-out" lesions in the flat and tubular bones. Some may appear as a discrete lytic lesion and remain as a solitary lesion. **(REF. 4, p. 1754)**

356. A. The diagnosis is sickle cell anemia. There is a biconcave appearance or configuration of the vertebral bodies, giving rise to a "fish mouth" appearance. Some sclerotic changes are seen. **(REF. 4, p. 850)**

357. E. Autoimmune hemolytic anemia is the most likely diagnosis. Spherocytosis is seen as well in burn victims, in microangiopathic hemolysis, and in congenital spherocytosis. **(REF. 2, p. 1650)**

358. C. A number of factors influence the rate and degree of hemoglobin S aggregation including concentration of S in the cell, cellular dehydration, and the length of time in deoxy conformation. **(REF. 1, p. 888)**

359. D. The patients with homozygous hemoglobin C disease have mild hemolysis, splenomegaly, target cells, and hemoglobin C crystals. **(REF. 1, p. 892)**

Diseases of the Blood / 143

360. A. In one class of beta thalassemia (beta plus) there is a mutation which affects processing of the beta globin messenger RNA precursor. **(REF. 1, p. 885)**

361. B. A moderately severe decrease in alpha chain production leads to the formation of very unstable four-beta chain tetramers that are useless in oxygen transport. **(REF. 1, p. 885)**

362. C. If the bone infarction occurs in proximity to a joint, an effusion can develop. The underlying pathology is a vasoocclusive phenomenon. **(REF. 1, p. 889)**

363. C. Both of these myeloproliferative disorders have findings associated with increased rates of white cell production and turnover, including serum uric acid and vitamin B_{12}. **(REF. 1, pp. 928, 939)**

364. C. Chronic myelogenous leukemia cells are thought to be clonal because the Philadelphia chromosome is present in several cell lines. Studies with G-6-PD isoenzymes show that polycythemia is also likely to be clonal. **(REF. 1, pp. 927, 938)**

365. D. Although CML is a form of leukemia, and all other leukemias frequently present with low platelets, CML and polycythemia as myeloproliferative disorders usually have elevated or normal platelet counts. **(REF. 1, pp. 928, 938)**

366. C. Myelofibrosis is usually present late in the course of CML but, rarely, acute myelofibrosis may occur early. Polythemia frequently terminates with myelofibrosis in the so-called "spent" phase. **(REF. 1, pp. 928, 940)**

367. E. In addition to the four symptoms cited, other neurologic symptoms include motor weakness, muscle atrophy, ptosis, facial palsy, and ileus. **(REF. 4, p. 1873)**

368. D. Hemoglobin S is characterized by hydrophobic

144 / Diseases of the Blood

bonding in the reduced state. Analysis of hemoglobin S has shown a substitution of valine for glutamine at position 6 of the beta chain. The resulting hemoglobin (hemoglobin S) runs slower than A on electrophoresis. (REF. 4, p. 837)

369. E. The renal concentrating defect and positive sickle prep are constant, but occlusive phenomena and hematuria may occur under stress. (REF. 4, p. 855)

370. E. All four statements are correct. The megaloblastic anemia of pregnancy is the most common of all folate-deficient states. Dilutional anemia and iron deficiency also occur in pregnancy. (REF. 4, p. 550)

371. B. This condition is usually associated with a positive Coombs' test using the baby's red blood cells and a positive indirect Coombs' test using the mother's serum. The mother is Rh negative and makes IgG antibodies against D positive cells of her baby. (REF. 4, p. 909)

372. A. Chronic infection does not occur in association with elevation of the serum iron-binding capacity. Iron in serum is bound to transferrin, a molecule which carries two atoms of iron per mole. (REF. 4, pp. 156, 610)

373. C. Decreased osmotic fragility is found in thalassemia minor and in iron deficiency anemia. Target cells and microcytes are resistant to osmotic swelling, whereas spherocytes are susceptible. (REF. 4, p. 747)

374. E. All the items listed are correct. Other categories of intravascular red cell destruction include erythrocyte fragmentation, autoimmune hemolytic anemias, and thermal injuries. (REF. 4, p. 501)

375. D. Hereditary persistence of hemoglobin F can be characterized as a benign genetic abnormality. Hemoglobin F is evenly distributed among red cells, unlike the increased F in other conditions. (REF. 4, p. 886)

Diseases of the Blood / 145

376. C. The spleen normally functions to pit nuclei and their fragments from red cells. **(REF. 4, p. 263)**

377. B. The dangers are that type A_2 may be mistyped as O and that O donors have high titers of anti-A and anti-B in their plasma. High titers of anti-A or anti-B are usually absorbed in the recipient's tissues, since A and B are represented on cells other than red cells. **(REF. 4, p. 492)**

378. B. The anemia is due to decreased globin chain production and to increased red cell destruction. Increased destruction stems from precipitated hemoglobin on the inner red cell surface. **(REF. 4, p. 872)**

379. B. Contact activation involves the intrinsic pathway and depends on Factor XII. Glass absorbs Factor XII to start the intrinsic pathway, a role played by collagen in vivo. **(REF. 4, p. 415)**

380. E. Extravascular hemolysis usually occurs in the liver, spleen, or other RE sites and liberates bilirubin unconjugated. **(REF. 4, p. 504)**

381. D. Spherocytosis is not associated with glucose-6-phosphate dehydrogenase deficiency. Spherocytes are characterized by normocytic hyperchromic indices with MCHC between 37 and 40%. **(REF. 4, p. 756)**

382. B. All mechanisms listed help to clear hemoglobin or heme from the plasma. Unconjugated bilirubin is not cleared by the kidney. **(REF. 4, p. 502)**

383. C. Bone marrow examination is most likely to show increased erythroid to myeloid ratio. Erythroid hyperplasia is common to all hemolytic anemias and may develop megaloblastic features unless folate is supplied. **(REF. 4, p. 504)**

384. E. Hypochromia would not be a change in the periphe-

146 / Diseases of the Blood

ral blood smear. Reticulocytes are large polychromatophilic cells that may have basophilic stippling. Normoblasts are released in brisk hemolysis. (REF. 4, p. 504)

385. E. Hemoglobinopathy is not a likely cause of anemia in this patient. Gastrointestinal bleeding from a duodenal ulcer; gastritis; or bleeding varices with iron deficiency are the commonest causes. (REF. 4, pp. 661, 668, 581)

386. B. Folate deficiency results from decreased intake and malabsorption. (REF. 4, p. 581)

387. A. Alcohol is directly toxic to dividing and maturing cells but may also affect neutrophil function. (REF. 4, p. 661)

388. D. The peripheral smear would not show increased platelet adhesiveness. The red cell changes may result from folate deficiency, associated liver disease, or plasma lipid concentration changes. (REF. 4, p. 581)

389. D. Coagulation Factors II, VII, X, and V would most likely be deficient. These are the factors that are synthesized in the liver, but V is not dependent on vitamin K. (REF. 4, p. 1210)

390. A. Polycythemia vera is less frequent in Negroes and more common in Jews. Males are more commonly affected and patients are usually middle-aged. (REF. 4, p. 1596)

391. E. Red cell mass is measured by ^{51}Cr-tagged red cells and the dilution method; plasma volume is measured by radioactive iodine-tagged albumin. (REF. 4, p. 1596)

392. B. In addition to radioactive phosphorus, alkylating agents such as chlorambucil are also used, and phlebotomy is used in most patients. (REF. 4, p. 1596)

393. D. Hemolytic crisis is not a complication. Vascular thrombosis is a hazard, which along with excessive hemorrhage, is relieved by phlebotomy. (REF. 4, p. 1596)

394. A. Normal arterial oxygen saturation is the most distinguishing feature. Secondary polycythemia may be caused by hypoxia or by erythropoietin-producing tumors. **(REF. 4, p. 1596)**

395. B. Thalassemia minor usually represents a heterozygous state and is often asymptomatic. **(REF. 4, p. 609)**

396. E. A serum iron determination would be most helpful. Iron stores in thalassemia are greatly increased, as in most chronic hemolytic anemias. **(REF. 4, p. 609)**

397. A. An increased amount of fetal A_2 hemoglobin would be expected. Since beta chains are decreased, the alpha chains combine with gamma and delta chains to make F and A_2. **(REF. 4, p. 614)**

398. C. The present treatment of choice is purely supportive. Care is taken to watch for anemia during intercurrent illness, due to aregenerative crises **(REF. 4, p. 891)**

399. D. Hemoglobin C characteristically produces targeting in the peripheral blood. Targeting is also seen in liver disease and may represent redundant membrane. **(REF. 4, p. 856)**

6. Diseases of the Kidneys: Fluids and Electrolytes

DIRECTIONS: Each of the questions or incomplete statements below is followed by five suggested answers or completions. Select the **one** that is **best** in each case.

---

400. All of the following substances are added to the urine by means of tubular secretion EXCEPT
    A. potassium
    B. hydrogen ion
    C. penicillin
    D. urea
    E. creatinine

401. Regarding nephroblastoma (Wilms' tumor)
    A. no treatment is available
    B. it occurs largely in adults
    C. it usually presents as distant metastasis
    D. it is often associated with hypertension
    E. it has the best prognosis in older patients

402. Acute glomerulonephritis may follow infection with
    A. type 12 group B α-hemolytic streptococci
    B. group A staphylococci
    C. group A α-hemolytic streptocci
    D. rickettsialpox
    E. *Escherichia coli* urinary tract sepsis

403. Which of the following urinary findings is most characteristic of acute glomerulonephritis?
 A. Proteinuria
 B. Microhematuria
 C. Granular casts
 D. Erythrocyte casts
 E. Hyaline casts

404. After recovery from acute nephritis, prophylactic therapy should include
 A. nothing
 B. penicillin G by mouth
 C. benzathine penicillin G intramuscularly
 D. tetracycline
 E. sulfonamides

405. In the obligatory diuresis following relief of urinary obstruction, the urine is
 A. dilute and alkaline
 B. low in sodium
 C. concentrated
 D. acid
 E. none of the above

406. Chronic phenacetin ingestion may lead to
 A. glomerulosclerosis
 B. papillary necrosis
 C. cortical necrosis
 D. tubular necrosis
 E. nephrolithiasis

407. Renal vein thrombosis may be caused by all of the following EXCEPT
 A. hypernephroma
 B. periarteritis
 C. severe dehydration
 D. abdominal injury
 E. glomerulonephritis

150 / Diseases of the Kidneys: Fluids and Electrolytes

408. Acute glomerulonephritis may be mimicked by all of the following EXCEPT
   A. periarteritis nodosa
   B. allergic purpura
   C. subacute bacterial endocarditis
   D. pyelonephritis
   E. lupus erythematosus

409. The nephrotic syndrome is characterized by all of the following signs EXCEPT
   A. edema
   B. proteinuria
   C. hypoalbuminemia
   D. hyperlipemia
   E. hypertension

410. Malignant hypertension may occur during the course of all the following EXCEPT
   A. pyelonephritis
   B. amyloidosis
   C. periarteritis nodosa
   D. primary nephrosclerosis
   E. pheochromocytoma

411. The kidney in sickle cell anemia is characterized by
   A. an inability to acidify the urine
   B. a decrease in glomerular filtration
   C. an inability to concentrate the urine
   D. pyuria
   E. a salt-losing state

412. During the recovery period of acute tubular necrosis the blood urea
   A. rises for several days
   B. falls immediately
   C. falls but creatinine rises
   D. remains low
   E. remains high

413. Cystinuria is a congenital disorder characterized by decreased tubular reabsorption of all of the following EXCEPT
    A. cystine
    B. arginine
    C. ornithine
    D. valine
    E. lysine

414. In patients with gout, renal disease is often manifested by all of the following EXCEPT
    A. glomerulonephritis
    B. pyelonephritis
    C. urate crystals
    D. vascular sclerosis
    E. proteinuria

415. Hypercalcemia occurs in all of the following EXCEPT
    A. sarcoidosis
    B. multiple myeloma
    C. acute osteoporosis
    D. cirrhosis
    E. Burnett's syndrome

416. Intravenous pyelography must be performed with special caution in patients with
    A. hyperparathyroidism
    B. pyelonephritis
    C. nephrolithiasis
    D. hypernephroma
    E. multiple myeloma

417. Amyloidosis of the kidneys may be associated with all of the following EXCEPT
    A. leprosy
    B. hypertension
    C. retinitis
    D. ulcerative colitis
    E. hematuria

152 / Diseases of the Kidneys: Fluids and Electrolytes

418. Renal involvement in multiple myeloma is characterized by
    A. nitrogen retention
    B. hypertension
    C. retinitis
    D. edema
    E. hematuria

419. Eclampsia differs from preeclampsia by the presence of
    A. hypertension
    B. edema
    C. albuminuria
    D. convulsions
    E. pregnancy

420. Hematuria presenting as initial bleeding only, may be due to
    A. kidney tumor
    B. ureteral stone
    C. severe bladder hemorrhage
    D. urethral lesions
    E. none of the above

421. Papillary necrosis is prone to occur in
    A. diabetes mellitus
    B. glomerulonephritis
    C. pyelonephritis
    D. hypertension
    E. cortical necrosis

422. Magnesium deficiency may be seen in all of the following EXCEPT
    A. cerebellar hemangioma
    B. malabsorption syndromes
    C. chronic alcoholism
    D. long-term parenteral therapy
    E. diabetic acidosis

423. All of the following are true about orthostatic proteinuria EXCEPT
    A. it is more pronounced in lordosis
    B. it is aggravated by prolonged standing
    C. it manifests protein-free early morning urine
    D. it only occurs with renal parenchymal disease
    E. that up to 3 gm per liter are seen

424. The intravenous replacement of fluids lost through excessive sweating should consist of
    A. normal saline in 5% dextrose/water
    B. one-half normal saline in 5% dextrose/water
    C. 5% dextrose in water
    D. Ringer's lactated solution
    E. whole plasma

425. The chief cause of chyluria is
    A. filariasis
    B. hyperlipemia
    C. hypercholesterolemia
    D. lymphosarcoma
    E. rectovesical fistula

426. Hypernephroma has been associated with all of the following EXCEPT
    A. polycythemia
    B. fever
    C. hematuria
    D. renal vein thrombosis
    E. high incidence of hypertension

427. Blood levels of all of the following rise in acute renal failure EXCEPT
    A. creatinine
    B. sodium
    C. potassium
    D. uric acid
    E. urea

428. Hypernatremia includes all of the following responses EXCEPT
   A. thirst
   B. decreased secretion of ADH
   C. movement of water out of cells
   D. decreased rate of sweating
   E. concentration of urine

429. The nephropathy of potassium depletion is most strikingly characterized by
   A. inability to concentrate urine
   B. inability to dilute urine
   C. erythrocyte casts
   D. granular casts
   E. renal potassium wasting

430. Hyperkalemia of acute renal failure may be treated by all of the following methods EXCEPT
   A. sodium cycle resin (Kayexalate)
   B. hypotonic saline
   C. intravenous glucose and insulin
   D. sodium bicarbonate
   E. calcium chloride

431. The major intracellular cation is
   A. potassium
   B. sodium
   C. magnesium
   D. calcium
   E. phosphate

432. Inappropriate secretion of antidiuretic hormone may be associated with
    A. massive edema
    B. hypernatremia
    C. dehydration
    D. urine osmolality that is inappropriately low
    E. benign intrathoracic lesions

433. Sympathetic innervation to the bladder is most probably concerned with
    A. closure of the bladder neck during ejaculation
    B. sensation
    C. voluntary micturition
    D. relaxation of peritoneal muscles
    E. opening of the bladder neck

434. The largest volume of water is reabsorbed in the nephron at the
    A. collecting ducts
    B. proximal convolution
    C. distal convolution
    D. ascending loop of Henle
    E. desending loop of Henle

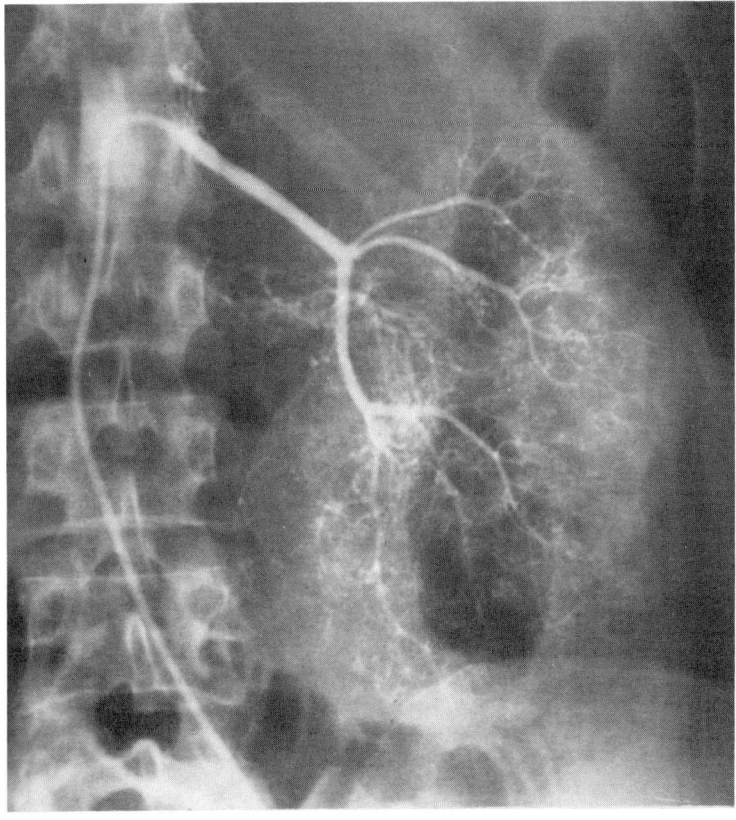

Figure 6.1

435. Figure 6.1 is a selective renal arteriogram done on a 64-year-old male who was admitted for hematuria after slipping on an icy pavement. What is your diagnosis?
   A. Renal cell carcinoma
   B. Kidney contusion and laceration
   C. Transitional cell carcinoma
   D. Renal hamartoma
   E. Renal hemangioma

DIRECTIONS: Each group of questions below consists of a list of lettered headings followed by a list of numbered words, phrases or statements. For **each** numbered word, phrase or statement, select the **one** lettered heading that is most closely associated with it. Each lettered heading may be selected once, more than once, or not at all.

    A. Metabolic acidosis
    B. Metabolic alkalosis
    C. Respiratory acidosis
    D. Respiratory alkalosis

436. Diarrhea leads to significant bicarbonate loss with a normal anion gap

437. Acute onset leads to somnolence, confusion, and ultimately, CO_2 narcosis

438. Can result from primary hyperaldosteronism because of renal bicarbonate generation

439. May be associated with isoniazid toxicity in which oxygen utilization by tissues is thought to be impaired

440. May occur acutely as a result of anxiety or salicylism

158 / Diseases of the Kidneys: Fluids and Electrolytes

DIRECTIONS: For each of the questions or incomplete statements below, **one** or **more** of the answers or completions is correct. Select

- **A** if only *1, 2 and 3* are correct,
- **B** if only *1 and 3* are correct,
- **C** if only *2 and 4* are correct,
- **D** if only *4* is correct,
- **E** if *all* are correct.

441. Conditions associated with increased urinary tract infections include
    1. anemia
    2. pregnancy
    3. exercise
    4. diabetes mellitus

442. Causes of rapidly progressive (subacute) glomerulonephritis include
    1. bacterial endocarditis
    2. Goodpasture's syndrome
    3. lupus erythematosus
    4. poststreptococcal disease

443. Diseases associated with the nephrotic syndrome include
    1. sickle cell disease
    2. medullary sponge kidneys
    3. radiation nephritis
    4. amyloid disease

444. Which of the following blood studies is seen in the nephrotic syndrome?
    1. Elevated cholesterol
    2. Elevated triglycerides
    3. Elevated phospholipids
    4. Low beta-lipoproteins

445. Polyuria is commonly seen in
1. hypercalcemia
2. glycosuria
3. hypokalemia
4. hyperkalemia

446. Which of the following is associated with toxemia of pregnancy?
1. Twin pregnancies
2. Second or third pregnancies
3. Hydatidiform moles
4. Youth of the gravid person

447. Which of the following is true of polycystic kidney disease?
1. It frequently affects only one kidney
2. Pregnancy aggravates the disease
3. Episodic oliguria is common
4. Marsupialization of cysts does not prolong life

448. Which of the following is associated with renal lithiasis?
1. Cystinuria
2. Hereditary glycinuria
3. Primary hyperoxaluria
4. Sarcoidosis

449. The presence of antidiuretic hormone causes increased permeability to water in the
1. glomerulus
2. distal convolution
3. proximal convolution
4. collecting duct

450. In azotemic patients, restriction of salt is wise
1. in congestive heart failure
2. with oliguria
3. with edema
4. at all times

Directions Summarized				
A	B	C	D	E
1,2,3 only	1,3 only	2,4 only	4 only	All are correct

451. Complications of acute renal failure include
    1. potassium intoxication
    2. pulmonary edema
    3. diastolic hypertension
    4. infections

452. Sudden deterioration of renal function in a diabetic should lead one to the diagnosis of
    1. acute pyelonephritis
    2. chronic pyelonephritis
    3. renal calculi
    4. papillary necrosis

6. Diseases of the Kidneys: Fluids and Electrolytes Answers and Comments

400. D. The clearance of urea, although partly determined by tubular process, is a rough indication of GFR. **(REF. 2, p. 1283)**

401. D. Wilms' tumor is often associated with hypertension. Actinomycin D and radiotherapy have given a five-year survival of 60% to 70%, with best results in children under age 2. **(REF. 2, p. 1356)**

402. C. Symptoms of acute glomerulonephritis do not usually develop until 7 to 20 days after the group A α-hemolytic streptococcal infection. **(REF. 1, p. 521)**

403. D. Granular and erythrocyte casts are both present, but the latter indicate bleeding from the glomerulus and are most characteristically seen. **(REF. 1, p. 521)**

404. A. It has not been convincingly shown that any form of treatment alters the course of the glomerular lesion. **(REF. 1, p. 521)**

405. A. The urine is dilute and alkaline and contains much sodium. The large volume is due in part to osmotic diuresis following urea accumulation. **(REF. 2, p. 1328)**

406. B. Chronic phenacetin ingestion may lead to papillar necrosis. Satisfactory understanding of the pathogenesis is lacking, but sensitivity reactions or industrial contaminants have been suggested. **(REF. 1, p. 543)**

407. E. Renal vein thrombosis is not caused by glomerulonephritis. In addition to those listed, other causes of renal vein thrombosis include metastases to retroperitoneal nodes, thrombophlebitis of the legs, congestive heart failure, and advanced renal disease. **(REF. 2, p. 1341)**

162 / Diseases of the Kidneys: Fluids and Electrolytes

408. D. Pyelonephritis does not mimic acute glomerulonephritis. The characteristic elevation and subsequent fall of the antistreptolysin O titer is excellent evidence for a preceding strep infection. **(REF. 2, p. 1327)**

409. E. The blood pressure is often normal, and the heart is not enlarged. **(REF. 2, p. 1315)**

410. B. Malignant hypertension does not characteristically occur during the course of amyloidosis. Malignant hypertension is characterized by severe headache, vomiting, visual disturbances, convulsions and stupor, which are signs of hypertensive encephalopathy. **(REF. 2, p. 1177)**

411. C. In sickle cell anemia the kidney is characterized by an inablity to concentrate the urine. Papillary necrosis may also occur in patients with homozygous sickle cell disease or sickle cell trait. **(REF. 2, pp. 1341, 1548)**

412. A. The BUN rises until excretion of urea exceeds its production, usually several days after urine output rises. **(REF. 1, p. 494)**

413. D. Cystinuria is a genetic disorder characterized by continued excessive excretion of the dibasic amino acid, cystine. **(REF. 2, pp. 471, 1347)**

414. A. In patients with gout, renal disease is not manifested by glomerulonephritis. Twenty percent to 40% of patients show albuminuria, which is rarely heavy in quantity and usually intermittent. **(REF. 2, pp. 481, 1335)**

415. D. Hypercalcemia leads to polyuria, polydypsia, and dehydration, or to nephrolithiasis; it does not occur in cirrhosis. **(REF. 2, p. 1336)**

416. E. Danger of acute renal failure after IVP has led to caution, especially in patients with multiple myeloma. The patient should not be dehydrated if the IVP is necessary. **(REF. 2, p. 1281)**

417. E. Amyloidosis of the kidneys docs not cause hematuria. Amyloidosis is commonly encountered as a complication of chronic suppuration, and causes of amyloidosis include osteomyelitis and tuberculosis. **(REF. 2, p. 1324)**

418. A. Nitrogen retention is characteristic of renal involvement in multiple myeloma. Hypercalcemia may produce transient or irreversible renal damage as do amyloid and myeloma cell infiltrates. **(REF. 2, p. 1837)**

419. D. Eclampsia differs from preeclampsia by the presence of convulsions. The most common histologic finding in the kidneys in eclampsia is marked swelling of the endothelial and epithelial cells of the glomeruli. **(REF. 2, p. 1342)**

420. D. Urethral lesions may cause hematuria that presents as initial bleeding only. Investigation of hematuria includes urinalysis, hematologic evaluation, radiologic evaluation, cystoscopy, and renal biopsy. **(REF. 2, pp. 216, 1285)**

421. A. Papillary necrosis is prone to occur in diabetes mellitus. It is also seen in sickle cell disease, chronic alcoholism, and vascular disease. **(REF. 2, p. 1332)**

422. A. Magnesium deficiency is usually accompanied by hypocalcemia, and it is not seen in cerebellar hemangioma. **(REF. 2, p. 1842)**

423. D. Orthostatic proteinuria occurs in many conditions and not only with renal parenchymal disease. Perhaps three-quarters of adolescents and young adults have proteinuria on prolonged standing or strenuous exercise. **(REF. 2, p. 1319)**

424. B. The loss of sweat contributes to a deficit of water in excess of salt loss; therefore, fluid replacement should consist of rb 1/2 normal saline in 5% dextrose/water. **(REF. 2, p. 436)**

425. A. Filariasis is the chief cause of chyluria. Obstruction between the abdominal lymphatics and the thoracic duct produces lymph varices in the kidney. **(REF. 2, p. 897)**

164 / Diseases of the Kidneys: Fluids and Electrolytes

426. E. Hypernephroma is not associated with a high incidence of hypertension. Hematuria, flank pain, and abdominal mass is the classical presentation, but metastases may be the first sign. **(REF. 2, p. 1355)**

427. B. Blood levels of sodium do not rise in acute renal failure. Patients with acute tubular necrosis do spontaneously excrete a moderately high percentage of filtered water and filtered sodium. **(REF. 1, p. 494)**

428. B. Decreased secretion of ADH is not a response in hypernatremia. Hypernatremia is the chemical expression of water deficit, and the adjustments in physiology retain or acquire water. **(REF. 2, p. 437)**

429. A. Inability to concentrate urine persists with dehydration; however, diluting ability is usually well preserved. **(REF. 1, p. 561)**

430. B. Hypotonic saline is not a treatment for hyperkalemia of acute renal failure. Intravenous glucose and insulin is used if marked hyperkalemia is present when the patient is first seen. **(REF. 1, p. 499)**

431. A. The difference between total tissue potassium and the quantity in the extracellular phase represents the intracellular amount. **(REF. 2, p. 436)**

432. E. Intrathoracic lesions may be benign or malignant, and the latter may secrete a substance similar to lysine vasopressin. **(REF. 2, p. 1684)**

433. A. Sympathetic innervation has little effect on bladder function, which is largely controlled by parasympathetics. **(REF. 2, p. 222)**

434. B. The largest volume of water is reabsorbed in the nephron at the proximal convolution. Maximally concentrated urine depends on ADH, which allows distal convoluted tubes and collecting ducts to become permeable to water. **(REF. 2, p. 217)**

435. A. The diagnosis is renal cell carcinoma. There is marked hypervascularity of the left kidney. The arteries are irregular and tortuous, following a random distribution. There are small vessels within the renal vein which indicate the blood supply of the neoplastic thrombosis involving the renal vein. The kidney is enlarged and abnormally bulbous in the lower pole. **(REF. 2, p. 1355)**

436. A. The anion gap is calculated as the sodium concentration minus the chloride plus the bicarbonate concentration. Other causes of bicarbonate loss with normal anion gap include proximal renal tubular acidosis and primary hyperparathyroidism. **(REF. 1, pp. 489, 490)**

437. C. Causes of acute respiratory acidosis include narcotic overdose, myasthenia gravis, airway obstruction, and trauma to the chest. **(REF. 1, pp. 493, 494)**

438. B. The disorder can occur in volume-expanded patients in which the alkalosis is unresponsive to sodium chloride loading, as in primary hyperaldosteronism or volume contraction with secondary hyperaldosteronism. **(REF. 1, p. 492)**

439. A. Impaired oxygen utilization leads to lactic acidosis, accumulation of lactate, and increased anion gap. **(REF. 1, p. 490)**

440. D. During acute hyperventilation, plasma bicarbonate concentrations fall by approximately 3 mEq per litre when the arterial pressure of CO_2 falls to about 25 mmHg. **(REF. 1, p. 494)**

441. C. Pregnancy and diabetes mellitus are associated with increased urinary tract infections, which are more common in females and predisposed by obstruction, instrumentation, renal diseases, hypertension, and neurogenic bladder dysfunction. **(REF. 2, p. 1328)**

442. E. All of the conditions listed are causes of subacute glomerulonephritis. Abrupt onset and rapid progression are the rule, with bloody urine, anemia, oliguria, and azotemia. **(REF. 2, p. 1311)**

443. D. In addition to amyloid disease, other conditions associated with the nephrotic syndrome are secondary syphilis, malaria, and treatment with mercurial diuretics and gold salts. **(REF. 2, p. 1315)**

444. A. Low beta-lipoproteins are not seen in the nephrotic syndrome. One reason for elevated serum cholesterol is increased solubility in fatty serum; and hyperlipemia usually disappears with elimination of edema. **(REF. 2, p. 1315)**

445. A. Polyuria is commonly seen in hyperkalemia. Diabetes insipidus from hormonal or nephrogenic causes also produces polyuria. **(REF. 2, p. 219)**

446. B. Twin pregnancies and hydatidiform moles are associated with toxemia of pregnancy. It also occurs in women pregnant for the first time, and in those over 35 years of age. **(REF. 2, p. 1342)**

447. D. Marsupialization of cysts does not prolong life in polycystic kidney disease. Renal transplantation is becoming an alternative form of therapy. **(REF. 2, p. 1343)**

448. E. All four conditions are associated with renal lithiasis. Cystinuria is a congenital disorder associated with decreased tubular resorption of cystine, arginine, ornithine, and lysine. **(REF. 2, p. 1349)**

449. C. The formation of maximally concentrated urine depends on the presence of antidiuretic hormone, which causes increased permeability to water in the distal convolution and the collecting duct. **(REF. 2, p. 1686)**

450. A. In azotemic patients with oliguria, salt and water intake produces circulatory congestion, and pulmonary edema is not relieved by digitalis. **(REF. 2, p. 1295)**

451. E. All four conditions listed are complications of acute renal failure. Complete anuria for more than 48 hours should suggest obstruction, bilateral renal arterial emboli, or thrombosis. **(REF. 2, p. 1295)**

452. D. Severe infection of the renal pyramids in association with vascular disease or obstruction leads to papillary necrosis. **(REF. 2, p. 1315)**

7. Diseases of Nutrition, Metabolism, and Endocrines

DIRECTIONS: Each of the questions or incomplete statements below is followed by five suggested answers or completions. Select the **one** that is **best** in each case.

453. The most common cause of hypothyroidism in the adult is
    A. trauma
    B. radioactive iodine ingestion
    C. primary hypothyroidism
    D. parathyroid surgery
    E. antithyroid chemicals

454. The earliest clinical manifestation of Sheehan's syndrome is
    A. failure to resume a normal menstrual cycle
    B. failure to regain normal strength and vigor following delivery
    C. loss of libido
    D. early mammary involution and failure to lactate
    E. adrenal insufficiency

455. All of the following are characteristics of panhypopituitarism EXCEPT
    A. occurrence of myxedema
    B. decreased melanin pigmentation
    C. emaciation and cachexia
    D. loss of axillary and pubic hairs
    E. moderate normocytic and normochromic anemia

456. Proinsulin can best be characterized as
    A. smaller than insulin
    B. a double helix
    C. immunologically similar to insulin
    D. completely inactive
    E. more active than insulin

457. Factors in the pathogenesis of diabetic ketoacidosis include all of the following EXCEPT
    A. reduced insulin action
    B. increased catecholamines
    C. increased glucosteroids
    D. increased growth hormone
    E. increased renin

458. In the human menstrual cycle, follicle-stimulating hormone can be said to
    A. cause ovulation
    B. encourage progesterone secretion
    C. cause the secretory phase of the uterine mucosa
    D. inhibit estrogen secretion
    E. encourage maturation of the follicle

459. The major steroid hormone regulating corticotrophin secretion is
    A. desoxycortisol
    B. cortisone
    C. cortol
    D. aldosterone
    E. cortisol

170 / Diseases of Nutrition, Metabolism, and Endocrines

460. Once lactation has developed, its maintenance depends on continued secretion of
   A. prolactin
   B. ACTII
   C. estrogen
   D. progesterone
   E. prolactin inhibiting factor

461. Findings in hyperparathyroidism include all of the following EXCEPT
   A. renal colic
   B. bone pain
   C. gastrointestinal symptoms
   D. mental confusion
   E. dyspnea

462. The most common cause of hypoparathyroidism is
   A. idopathic
   B. familial
   C. postradiation
   D. end organ resistance
   E. surgical removal

463. In adrenocortical insufficiency
   A. the skin is shiny and pale
   B. a diabetic glucose tolerance is characteristic
   C. water diuresis is impaired
   D. the urinary steroids are high
   E. none of the above

464. In thyrotoxicosis during pregnancy the best time for I^{131} therapy is
   A. the last trimester
   B. the second trimester
   C. the third trimester
   D. no special time
   E. none of the above

Diseases of Nutrition, Metabolism, and Endocrines / 171

465. Reducing substance may be found in the urine in all of the following conditions EXCEPT
    A. renal glycosuria
    B. pentosuria
    C. fructosuria
    D. oxalosis
    E. renal damage secondary to nephrotoxic agents

466. Patients with hepatic porphyria should avoid
    A. chlorpromazine
    B. barbiturates
    C. a high calcium diet
    D. narcotics
    E. steroids

467. Porphobilinogen is found in the urine of patients with
    A. intermittent acute porphyria
    B. erythropoietic porphyria
    C. porphyria cutanea tarda
    D. coproporphyria
    E. hemolytic anemia

468. Starvation of an obese subject for three weeks leads to
    A. the same glucose level as normals
    B. severe hypoglycemia
    C. decreased uric acid formation
    D. severe hyperglycemia
    E. blood glucose levels above the hypoglycemic level but below normal

469. Precipitating factors in acute gouty arthritis include all of the following EXCEPT
    A. alcohol
    B. high purine food
    C. roentgen therapy
    D. surgical procedure
    E. ACTH

Diseases of Nutrition, Metabolism, and Endocrines

470. The diagnosis of congenital galactosemia is suspected by finding
   A. increased glucose in the urine
   B. increased reducing substance, other than glucose, in the urine
   C. an autosomal dominant family history
   D. response to gluten-free diet
   E. hemolytic anemia

471. Tay-Sachs disease is characterized by all of the following EXCEPT
   A. glycogen storage
   B. ganglioside accumulation
   C. spasticity
   D. macular degeneration
   E. ballooning of cerebral ganglion cells

472. The characteristic neurologic findings in amyloidosis include
   A. peripheral motor and sensor neuropathy
   B. spinal cord compression in the lumbar region
   C. spinal cord compression in the thoracic region
   D. a peripheral neuropathy associated with cerebral manifestations
   E. a Guillain-Barré-type syndrome

473. One finds increased levels of 5-hydroxyindoleacetic acid in the urine in
   A. phenylketonuria
   B. alkaptonuria
   C. malignant melanoma
   D. carcinoid syndrome
   E. disseminated carcinomatosis

474. Carcinoid syndrome is characterized by all of the following EXCEPT
   A. valvular heart disease
   B. asthma
   C. hypertension
   D. diarrhea
   E. cyanosis

Diseases of Nutrition, Metabolism, and Endocrines / 173

475. Familial hyperbetalipoproteinemia (type II hyperlipoproteinemia) is characterized by
   A. milky serum
   B. severe diabetes
   C. aggravation with ingestion of polyunsaturated fats
   D. an increased incidence of coronary artery disease
   E. high serum triglycerides

476. The syndrome of congenital absence of beta-lipoproteins includes all of the following EXCEPT
   A. ataxic neuropathy
   B. crenated red blood cells (acanthocytosis)
   C. renal disease
   D. hypocholesterolemia
   E. retinopathy

477. An adult patient with hepatosplenomegaly and large reticulated cells in the bone marrow containing glucocerebrosides can be diagnosed as having
   A. metachromatic leukodystrophy
   B. Gaucher's disease
   C. reticulum cell sarcoma associated with diabetes
   D. glycogen storage disease
   E. familial hyperchylomicronemia

478. Diagnostic criteria for impaired thyroglobulin synthesis include all of the following EXCEPT
   A. goiter
   B. hypothyroid
   C. low radioiodine uptake
   D. presence of colloid spaces
   E. exclusion of other defects

479. Glycogen storage diseases
   A. do not affect the liver
   B. may cause xanthomas
   C. are always autosomal dominant
   D. are due to a single enzyme defect
   E. are corrected by surgery

174 / Diseases of Nutrition, Metabolism, and Endocrines

480. Cystinuria is commonly associated with
    A. severe mental retardation
    B. homocystinuria
    C. hexagonal crystals in the urine
    D. malnutrition due to urine loss of cystine
    E. hydrocephalus

481. The treatment of diabetic nephropathy is
    A. low insulin dosage
    B. oral hypoglycemic agents
    C. intermittent peritoneal dialysis
    D. complete control of diabetes
    E. none of the above

482. Magnesium deficiency may be seen in all of the following EXCEPT
    A. alcoholism
    B. chronic malabsorption
    C. diabetes mellitus
    D. kwashiorkor
    E. hypervitaminosis E

483. The syndrome of hepatomegaly, splenomegaly, leukopenia, anemia, periosteal changes, sparse and coarse hair, and increased serum lipids occurs in chronic
    A. vitamin D intoxication
    B. vitamin D deficiency
    C. vitamin A deficiency
    D. vitamin A intoxication
    E. acarotenemia

484. Which of the following is NOT true about dietary fat?
    A. It furnishes more calories per gram than carbohydrate
    B. Polyunsaturated fatty acids lower cholesterol
    C. Polyunsaturated fatty acids are nonessential nutrients
    D. Food fat aids vitamin absorption
    E. Medium chain fatty acids enter the portal tract directly

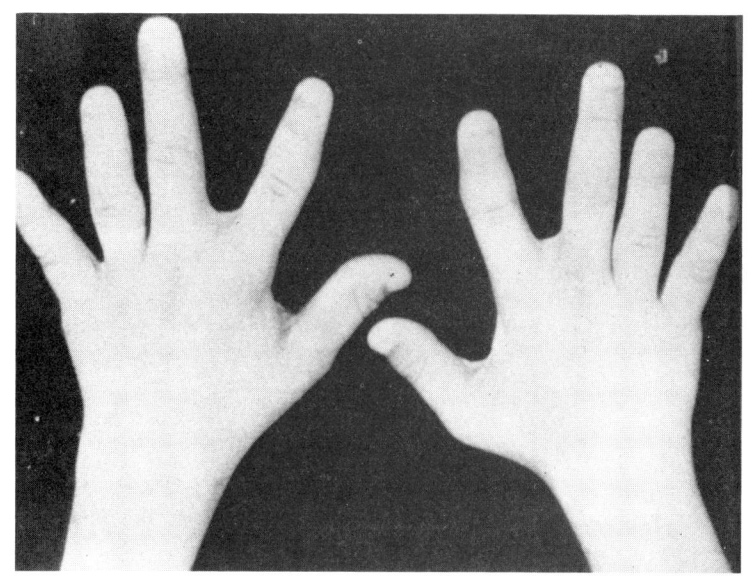

Diseases of Nutrition, Metabolism, and Endocrines / 175

Figure 7.1

485. The patient whose hands are shown in Figure 7.1 is mentally retarded with a short stocky build. What is the most likely diagnosis?
    A. Achondroplastic dwarf
    B. Down's syndrome
    C. Kleinfelter's syndrome
    D. Pseudohypoparathyroidism
    E. Turner's syndrome

486. Which of the following laboratory values is the above patient likely to show?
    A. Hypercalcemia, hypophosphatemia
    B. Hypocalcemia, low parathormone
    C. Hypocalcemia, high parathormone
    D. Hypocalcemia, hypophosphatemia
    E. Hyperphosphatemia, low parathormone

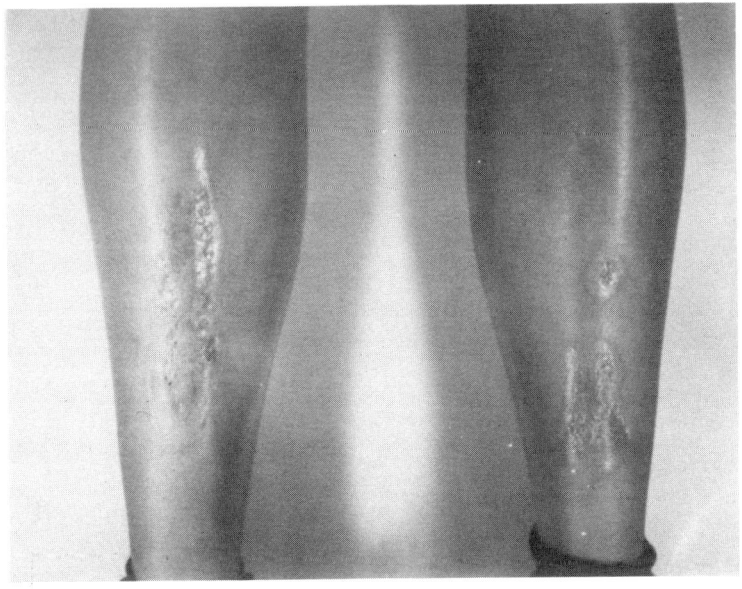

176 / Diseases of Nutrition, Metabolism, and Endocrines

Figure 7.2

487. A 28-year-old woman with diabetes has the leg lesions shown in Figure 7.2. What is the most likely diagnosis?
   A. Eruptive xanthomas
   B. Necrobiosis lipoidica diabeticorum
   C. Gangrene
   D. Staphylococcal infection
   E. Erythema nodosum

488. Allopurinol is useful in the prevention of gout because of which of the following mechanisms of action?
   A. Inhibition of xanthine oxidase
   B. Solubilization of uric acid
   C. Reactivity with hypoxanthine
   D. Anti-inflammatory effect on joint tissue
   E. Increased renal tubular secretion of uric acid

Diseases of Nutrition, Metabolism, and Endocrines / 177

489. Hypomagnesemia may result in all of the following EXCEPT
  A. lethargy
  B. neuromuscular irritability
  C. anorexia
  D. tachyarrhythmias
  E. hyperkalemia

490. A 22-year-old man with arm span greater than height, subluxed lenses, flattened corneas, and dilation of the aortic ring is most likely to have
  A. Ehlers-Danlos syndrome
  B. Marfan's syndrome
  C. Werner's syndrome
  D. Laurence-Moon-Biedl syndrome
  E. Hunter's syndrome

491. Which of the following hypothalamic substances is inhibitory in its action?
  A. Corticotropin-releasing factor
  B. Thyrotropin-releasing factor
  C. Somatostatin
  D. Growth hormone-releasing factor
  E. Prolactin-releasing factor

492. Patients with chromophobic pituitary tumors are most likely to initially complain to their doctors of
  A. amenorrhea or impotence
  B. galactorrhea
  C. urinary frequency
  D. visual complaints
  E. inappropriate cold intolerance

493. Which of the following drugs suppresses the release of antidiuretic hormone?
  A. Diphenylhydantoin
  B. Cyclophosphamide
  C. Barbiturates
  D. Nicotine
  E. Morphine

Diseases of Nutrition, Metabolism, and Endocrines

DIRECTIONS: Each group of questions below consists of five lettered headings followed by a list of numbered words, phrases, or statements. For **each** numbered word, phrase or statement, select the **one** lettered heading that is most closely associated with it. Each lettered heading may be selected once, more than once, or not at all.

- A. Addison's disease
- B. Pheochromocytoma
- C. Aldosteronism
- D. Hyperparathyroidism
- E. Failure to secrete

494. Hyponatremia

495. Glycosuria

496. Paroxysmal hypertension

497. Elevated BMR

498. Periodic paralysis

- A. Palmar plane xanthomas
- B. Triglycerides greater than 1000
- C. Subcutaneous extensor tendon xanthomas
- D. Low serum cholesterol
- E. Cholesterol normal

499. Hyperchylomicronemia

500. Hyperbetalipoproteinemia

501. Type III hyperlipoproteinemia

502. Hyperprebetalipoproteinemia

503. Hyperglyceridemia

DIRECTIONS: Each set of lettered headings below is followed by a list of numbered words or phrases. For each numbered word or phrase select

    A if the item is associated with (A) *only,*
    B if the item is associated with (B) *only,*
    C if the item is associated with *both* (A) *and* (B),
    D if the item is associated with *neither* (A) *nor* (B).

    A. Diabetes mellitus (DM)
    B. Diabetes insipidus (DI)
    C. Both
    D. Neither

504. Polyuria and polydipsia

505. Not associated with renal disease

506. Does not occur as a result of tumors

507. Associated with a positive Hickey-Hare test

508. Related in some manner to obesity

    A. Type II hyperlipoproteinemia
    B. Type IV hyperlipoproteinemia
    C. Both
    D. Neither

509. Increased risk of heart disease

510. Subcutaneous xanthomas

511. Pattern seen in diabetes mellitus

512. Hyperchylomicronemia

513. Treatment with low carbohydrate

180 / Diseases of Nutrition, Metabolism, and Endocrines

DIRECTIONS: For each of the questions or incomplete statements below, **one** or **more** of the answers or completions given is correct. Select
- A if only *1, 2 and 3* are correct,
- B if only *1 and 3* are correct,
- C if only *2 and 4* are correct,
- D if only *4* is correct,
- E if *all* are correct.

514. The cardinal signs and symptoms of Addison's disease include
    1. hypertension
    2. hyperglycemic attacks
    3. increased heart size
    4. abnormal pigmentation

515. Cardiac changes observed in thyrotoxicosis may be
    1. systolic murmurs
    2. auricular fibrillation
    3. tachycardia
    4. cardiomegaly on x-ray

516. Biopsy of the thyroid may be useful in the diagnosis of
    1. chronic thyroiditis
    2. nontoxic multinodular goiter
    3. subacute thyroiditis
    4. malignant neoplasms

517. A pituitary tumor may be suspected by the finding of
    1. erosion of the bony walls of the sella turcica
    2. loss of vision due to pressure on the optic nerves
    3. frequent headaches
    4. loss of hearing due to pressure on the eighth nerve

Diseases of Nutrition, Metabolism, and Endocrines / 181

518. The release of vasopressin is controlled by
    1. hypertonicity of the blood perfusing the head
    2. phosphate levels in the renal plasma
    3. volume receptors in the left atrium and vascular areas
    4. cerebrospinal fluid pressure

519. Nonfunctioning nodules of the thyroid should be
    1. immediately treated by radical surgery
    2. treated with a large dose of I^{131}
    3. treated with a thyrotropin
    4. considered possibly malignant

520. The differential diagnosis of hypoglycemia includes
    1. excess growth hormone
    2. Cushing's disease
    3. thyrotoxicosis
    4. tumor of the pancreatic beta cells

521. Tests that measure the tubular reabsorption of phosphate are abnormal in
    1. diabetes mellitus
    2. hyperparathyroidism
    3. hyperthyroidism
    4. intrinsic renal disease with a BUN of 100 mg%

522. Which of the following are important signs or symptoms of acromegaly?
    1. Enlarged sella
    2. Pigmentation
    3. Hypermetabolism
    4. Soft tissue growth

523. Glucagon can be best described as a hormone that is
    1. secreted by the alpha cells of the pancreas
    2. a carbohydrate in structure
    3. effective in raising blood sugar levels
    4. antigenically similar to insulin

Diseases of Nutrition, Metabolism, and Endocrines

Directions Summarized				
A	B	C	D	E
1,2,3 only	1,3 only	2,4 only	4 only	All are correct

524. Hyperparathyroidism may be associated with
    1. the Zollinger-Ellison syndrome
    2. an adrenal adenoma
    3. acromegaly
    4. a testicular carcinoma

525. Administration of estrogen results in which of the following effects?
    1. Development of secondary sexual characteristics
    2. Development of the secretory phase of the endometrium
    3. Thickening of the vaginal mucosa with cornification
    4. A decrease of sebaceous gland activity

526. Feminizing adrenocortical tumors are
    1. usually benign
    2. associated with hypertension
    3. associated with an increase in the size of the phallus
    4. usually malignant

527. Excessive growth hormone affects the muscles by causing
    1. enlargement
    2. spasm
    3. weakness
    4. myositis

528. Vitamin D-resistant rickets is associated with
    1. hypophosphatemia
    2. increased calcium absorption
    3. osteomalacia
    4. osteoporosis

529. Diabetic ketosis is usually precipitated by
    1. infection
    2. surgical procedures or trauma
    3. acute myocardial infarction
    4. gastrointestinal disturbances with decreased food intake or vomiting

530. Gouty patients may have as associated diseases
    1. pernicious anemia
    2. obesity
    3. diabetes insipidus
    4. hypertriglyceridemia

531. In osteomalacia which of the following may occur?
    1. Bending of long bones
    2. Milkman's syndrome (pseudofractures)
    3. Absence of lamina dura
    4. Nephrocalcinosis

532. Complications of Paget's disease of the bone include
    1. renal calculi
    2. osteogenic sarcoma
    3. hypercalcemia
    4. secondary hyperparathyroidism

533. A deficiency of vitamin D can lead to
    1. decreased gastrointestinal absorption of calcium
    2. hypercalcemia
    3. decreased renal excretion of calcium
    4. decreased renal excretion of phosphorus

534. Ammonia levels in the blood are determined by
    1. protein catabolism
    2. amino-acid catabolism
    3. absorption from the gut
    4. hepatocellular function

Directions Summarized				
A	B	C	D	E
1,2,3 only	1,3 only	2,4 only	4 only	All are correct

535. In phenylketonuria the best treatment includes
    1. a gluten-free diet to age 12
    2. early detection by mass screening
    3. total elimination of phenylalanine from the diet
    4. long-term dietary control

536. The triad of Wilson's disease includes
    1. cirrhosis of the liver
    2. low ceruloplasmin
    3. signs of basal ganglia disease
    4. increased plasma copper

537. Phenylketonuria is treated by a diet low in
    1. phenylglycine
    2. 2-4 dinitrophenylhydrazine
    3. phenylhydrazine
    4. phenylalanine

538. Metabolic effects of insulin on adipose tissue
    1. accelerate transport of glucose
    2. decrease glucose phosphorylation
    3. decrease cyclic AMP
    4. decrease lipoprotein lipase

539. The management of patients with thyroid storm should include
    1. propylthiouracil
    2. hydrocortisone
    3. propranolol
    4. salicylates

540. Clinical signs of Addison's disease include
    1. weight loss
    2. lethargy
    3. hypotension
    4. skin pigmentation

541. Delayed adolescence in the male is usually due to
    1. inadequate diet
    2. pituitary tumor
    3. Leydig cell dysfunction
    4. normal variation

542. Response to hormone treatment of carcinoma of the breast is improved in which of the following situations?
    1. Metastases confined to liver
    2. Estrogen receptor present in tumor cell cytoplasm
    3. Patient more than five years premenopausal
    4. Disease-free interval in excess of two years

543. Which of the following represent increased risk factors for carcinoma of the breast?
    1. Maternal history of breast cancer
    2. Castration before age 40
    3. Late first pregnancy
    4. Long-term nursing

544. Primary carcinoid tumors may arise in the
    1. terminal ileum
    2. large bowel
    3. bronchus
    4. ovaries

186 / Diseases of Nutrition, Metabolism, and Endocrines

DIRECTIONS: This section consists of situations, each followed by a series of questions. Study each situation, and select the **one** best answer to each question following it.

CASE 1 (Questions 545–549): A healthy-appearing 30-year-old male was admitted with a one-year history of hypertension and polyuria. The physical examination was negative aside from hypertension. T waves were flat on EKG, and the only abnormal laboratory determination was a low potassium.

545. The triad of hypertension, hypokalemia, and polyuria in a healthy-appearing individual is characteristic of
   A. hypercorticism
   B. adult adrenogenital syndrome
   C. hyperaldosteronism
   D. familial hypokalemia

546. This condition is often associated with
   A. psychosis
   B. malignant hypertension
   C. hypokalemic alkalosis
   D. diabetic glucose tolerance curve
   E. pituitary tumor

547. These patients are always treated by
   A. adrenal suppression
   B. adrenal surgery
   C. pituitary irradiation
   D. adrenal radiation
   E. hypophysectomy

548. The pathology of this condition in the vast majority is
   A. a single, benign adenoma
   B. multiple, bilateral benign adenomas
   C. bilateral hyperplasia
   D. a malignant adenoma
   E. multiple endocrine adenomas

549. Which of the following, if present, would rule out this syndrome?
    A. Elevated serum sodium level
    B. Periodic paralysis
    C. Albuminuria
    D. Malignant hypertension with papilledema
    E. Paresthesias

CASE 2 (Questions 550-554): A 35-year-old obese female complains of recent weight loss in spite of a large appetite, vulvar pruritus, and waking up frequently at night to urinate.

550. The most likely diagnosis is
    A. diabetes mellitus
    B. diabetes insipidus
    C. vaginitis and cystitis
    D. myxedema
    E. pheochromocytoma

551. The diagnosis may be established by any of the following EXCEPT
    A. a urine glucose and acetone
    B. an insulin tolerance test
    C. a fasting blood sugar
    D. a glucose tolerance test
    E. a two-hour postprandial blood glucose

552. Eye examination might reveal any of the following EXCEPT
    A. central microaneurysms
    B. retinal exudates
    C. retinal hemorrhages
    D. retinitis proliferans
    E. open-angle glaucoma

188 / Diseases of Nutrition, Metabolism, and Endocrines

553. Which of the following renal diseases is this patient most likely to develop?
    A. Acute glomerulonephritis
    B. Obstructive uropathy
    C. Intercapillary glomerulosclerosis
    D. Renal infarction
    E. Polycystic kidneys

554. All of the following cutaneous manifestations may be found EXCEPT
    A. necrobiosis lipoidica
    B. xanthomas
    C. pyoderma gangrenosum
    D. candidiasis
    E. dermatophytosis

Diseases of Nutrition, Metabolism, and Endocrines / 189

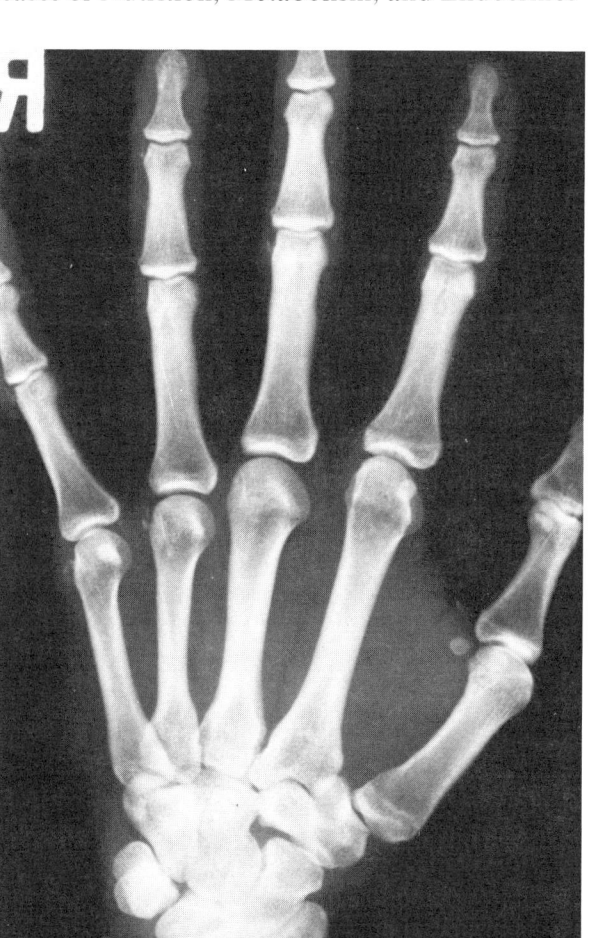

Figure 7.3

555. Figure 7.3 is the x-ray of a 35-year-old female with chronic renal disease complaining of pain in the hand after dialysis. What is your diagnosis?
    A. Scleroderma
    B. Gout
    C. Hyperparathyroidism
    D. Pseudogout
    E. Paget's disease

Case Work-up

	Normal	Patient
Plasma ACTH pg/ml	<150	<50
Plasma cortisol μg/ml	17	35
Urine 17-OH mg/24 hr	2-10	25
Urine 17-KS mg/24 hr	5-15	10
Urine 17-OH response to:		
ACTH IV	increase × 5	No response
Dexamethasone 0.5 mg	<3.0	No response
2.0 mg	<3.0	No response
Metyrapone 750 mg	increase × 2	No response

556. The case work-up shown above is of a 35-year-old woman presenting with hypertension, central obesity, and skin striae. The most likely diagnosis is
    A. adrenal hyperplasia secondary to hypothalamic dysfunction
    B. adrenal adenoma with complete autonomy
    C. exogenous steroids, iatrogenic
    D. pituitary tumor
    E. carcinoma of the adrenal

7. Diseases of Nutrition, Metabolism, and Endocrines Answers and Comments

453. C. Primary hypothyroidism is the most common cause of hypothyroidism in adults. Primary hypothyroidism is several times more common in women than in men and occurs most often between the ages of 40 and 60. **(REF.** 7, p. 217)

454. D. Postpartum hemorrhage with attendant shock and coagulation abnormalities is the precipitating cause of ischemic necrosis (Sheehan's syndrome), and early mammary involution and failure to lactate are the earliest clinical manifestations. **(REF.** 7, p. 93)

455. C. Patients with panhypopituitarism are found to have a normal distribution of body weight and are rarely cachectic or even undernourished. **(REF.** 7, p. 93)

456. C. Proinsulin is best characterized as immunologically similar to insulin. Proinsulin antiserum reacts with both insulin and proinsulin of different species. **(REF.** 7, p. 720)

457. E. Increased renin is not a pathogenetic factor. The other hormones, as well as glucagon, antagonize insulin in one of several ways, contributing to increased ketone bodies. **(REF.** 7, p. 806)

458. E. FSH is said to encourage maturation of the follicle in the human menstrual cycle. The cardinal hormonal change in phase one is a rise in FSH caused by a decrease in the level of estrogens and a waning activity of the corpus luteum. **(REF.** 7, p. 81)

459. E. Cortisol is the major steroid hormone regulating corticotrophin secretion. ACTH is one of the many hormones now known to act through the mediation of cyclic AMP. **(REF.** 7, p. 615)

192 / Diseases of Nutrition, Metabolism, and Endocrines

460. A. The hypothalamus may contain a prolactin-releasing factor that is released in response to suckling. **(REF. 7, p. 402)**

461. E. The first four signs listed are findings in hyperparathyroidism. Dyspnea is not usually seen. Most patients with hyperparathyroidism have a simple adenoma which functions autonomously, so that hormone is secreted with high calcium. **(REF. 7, p. 962)**

462. E. Surgical removal is the most common cause of hypoparathyroidism. When the glands or their blood vessels have merely been damaged and not removed, tissue often regenerates. **(REF. 7, p. 991)**

463. C. Water diuresis is impaired in adrenocortical insufficiency. Lack of aldosterone also favors the development of hyperkalemia and mild acidosis. **(REF. 7, p. 1043)**

464. E. Radioactivity is harmful to the developing fetus, and iodine may induce goiter in the fetus. **(REF. 7, p. 197)**

465. D. Reducing substance is not present in the urine in oxalosis. Fructosuria is an autosomal recessive condition. Adults may notice dyspepsia and anxiety with fructose ingestion. **(REF. 7, p. 860)**

466. B. In patients with hepatic porphyria, oral phenothiazines may be used for abdominal or muscle pains, and Demerol may also be used, but barbiturates should be avoided. **(REF. 1, p. 1122)**

467. A. Porphobilinogen is found in the urine of patients with intermittent acute porphyria. It is a colorless compound giving a red complex with Ehrlich aldehyde reagent in the Watson-Schwartz test. **(REF. 1, p. 1123)**

468. E. Starvation of an obese subject for three weeks leads to blood glucose levels above the hypoglycemic level but below normal. Severely malnourished individuals may also be prone to develop hypoglycemia after minor stress. **(REF. 9, p. 359)**

469. E. ACTH is not a precipitating factor in acute gouty arthritis. Some events such as starvation and alcohol increase urate levels by inhibition of renal urate excretion. **(REF.** 1, p. 1112)

470. B. The diagnosis is suspected by finding increased reducing substance, other than glucose, in the urine. Damage is produced by a block in the metabolism of galactose-1-phosphate, resulting in inhibition of glucose release from glycogen. **(REF.** 9, p. 370)

471. A. Glycogen storage is not characteristic of Tay-Sachs disease. Ganglioside accumulation can now be diagnosed by decreased hexosaminidase in peripheral leukocytes. **(REF.** 11, p. 852)

472. A. In addition to peripheral motor and sensory neuropathy, cardiac involvement, tongue enlargement, gastrointestinal manifestations, and carpal tunnel syndrome are also seen in amyloidosis. **(REF.** 1, p. 2162)

473. D. Carcinoid syndrome is characterized by increased levels of 5-hydroxyindoleacetic acid. The syndrome occurs in relation to malignant tumors which have metastasized, usually with hepatic implants. **(REF.** 1, p. 1312)

474. C. Hypertension is not a characteristic of carcinoid syndrome. Diarrhea may be recurrent, and mild to explosive, with abdominal pain, bloating, and severe tenesmus. **(REF.** 1, p. 1312)

475. D. In type II hyperlipoproteinemia there is an increased incidence of coronary artery disease, and hypercholesterolemia occurs along with tuberous xanthomas, arcus senilis, and atheromas. **(REF.** 9, p. 441)

476. C. In congenital absence of beta-lipoproteins there is an inability to manufacture the beta globulin required for beta-lipoprotein formation. Renal disease is not associated with this syndrome. **(REF.** 9, p. 411)

194 / Diseases of Nutrition, Metabolism, and Endocrines

477. B. The diagnosis is Gaucher's disease. The glucocerebrosides are derived from lipid catabolites from the membranes of senescent leukocytes and erythrocytes. **(REF. 9, p. 526)** *Skin pigmentation, skeletal lesions and pingueculae Autosomal recessive. Glucocerebrosidase lack. Splenectomy for pancytopenia.*

478. C. In impaired thyroglobulin synthesis, radioiodine uptake is normal or high and no thyroglobulin is found on thyroid biopsy. **(REF. 11, p. 226)**

479. B. Xanthomas may be caused by glycogen storage diseases. There are at least eight types of glycogen storage diseases, each caused by a different enzymatic abnormality. **(REF. 11, p. 137)**

480. C. Cystinuria is commonly associated with hexagonal crystals in the urine. Cystine, lysine, arginine, and ornithine are excreted in great excess by patients homozygous for the disease. **(REF. 9, p. 623)**

481. E. None of the treatments cited is used in diabetic nephropathy. Treatment of intercurrent infection and chronic dialysis or transplant may be helpful. **(REF. 7, p. 794)**

482. E. Magnesium deficiency is not seen in hypervitaminosis E. Causes of magnesium deficiency also include milk diets in infants, the diuretic phase of acute tubular necrosis, chronic diuretic therapy, acute pancreatitis, and inappropriate ADH. **(REF. 1, p. 881)**

483. D. Symptoms of vitamin A intoxication occur in infants or adults ingesting from 75,000 to 500,000 international units of vitamin A. The prognosis is good when vitamin A intake ceases. **(REF. 2, p. 431)**

484. C. Unsaturated fatty acids such as arachidonic acid and linoleic acid are essential nutrients in infants. Vitamins A, D, E, and K are absorbed with food fat. **(REF. 2, p. 432)**

485. D. The deformity of the hands is due to short metacar-

Diseases of Nutrition, Metabolism, and Endocrines / 195

pals. Other deformities include short metatarsals, round facies, and thickening of the calvarium. **(REF.** 1, p. 1301)

486. C. The findings of hypocalcemia and hyperphosphatemia are the same as in hypoparathyroidism, but the serum parathyroid hormone levels are appropriately increased. **(REF.** 1, p. 1301)

487. B. This lesion is more frequent in females and may antedate other clinical signs and symptoms of diabetes. **(REF.** 1, p. 1063)

488. A. Allopurinol inhibits the enzyme xanthine oxidase, resulting in decreased uric acid production. **(REF.** 1, p. 1110)

489. E. Magnesium deficiency results in hypokalemia beause of a tendency toward renal potassium wasting. **(REF.** 1, p. 1133)

490. B. Although the nature of the molecular defect is unknown, diminished type I collagen synthesis has been observed in tissue culture. **(REF.** 1, p. 1138)

491. C. Somatostatin inhibits TSH secretion as well as GH secretion and has widespread effects on secretion of gut hormones. **(REF.** 1, p. 1164)

492. D. Patients with pituitary tumors are most likely to seek aid because of visual or neurological symptoms, even though endocrine symptoms will be found to predate the presentation. **(REF.** 1, p. 1179)

493. A. Other drugs that suppress ADH release are alcohol, narcotic antagonists, and alpha-adrenergic agents. **(REF.** 1, p. 1196)

494. A. In Addison's disease, aldosterone deficiency also leads to weight loss, hypovolemia, hypotension, and prerenal azotemia. **(REF.** 7, p. 283)

196 / Diseases of Nutrition, Metabolism, and Endocrines

495. B. Increased fasting blood glucose level and abnormal results in the glucose tolerance test are attributable to catecholamine secretion. **(REF. 7, p. 543)**

496. B. In pheochromocytoma, hypertension may be sustained or paroxysmal, depending on the release pattern of norepinephrine into the blood. **(REF. 7, p. 543)**

497. B. In addition to an elevated BMR, other symptoms of pheochromocytoma include sweating, paroxysmal blanching or flushing, palpitation, tachycardia, and headache. **(REF. 7, p. 543)**

498. C. The diagnosis of aldosteronism is established by demonstrating elevated aldosterone secretion, subnormal plasma renin, and hypokalemia. Periodic paralysis may occur with aldosteronism. **(REF. 7, p. 277)**

499. B. In the familial form, the defect is believed to be a deficiency of lipoprotein lipase, with low release of this enzyme with heparin. **(REF. 2, p. 510)**

500. C. Subcutaneous xanthomas begin to appear at about age 20 and may involve achilles tendons, elbows, and tibial tuberosities. **(REF. 2, p. 510)**

501. A. In the rare familial form, raised, yellow plaques appear on palms and fingers, and reddish yellow xanthomas occur on the elbows. **(REF. 2, p. 510)**

502. E. Triglycerides are over 150 and are raised by alcohol intake, estrogens, stress, insulin, and physical activity. **(REF. 2, p. 510)**

503. B. Features include glucose intolerance, hyperinsulinemia, hyperuricemia, obesity, and excess ethanol intake. **(REF. 2, p. 510)**

504. C. In DM there is an obligatory osmotic diuresis, but in DI there is lack of water resorption in the tubules. **(REF. 1, pp. 1053, 1195)**

505. B. DM may develop Kimmelstiel-Wilson glomerulosclerosis, but DI affects tubular function only. **(REF. 1, pp. 1053, 1195)**

506. D. DM may follow pancreatic carcinoma, and DI may follow metastatic carcinoma, especially breast. **(REF. 1, pp. 1053, 1195)**

507. B. DI is associated with a positive Hickey-Hare test. Water restriction with observation of urine volume and concentration may be dangerous if dehydration occurs. **(REF. 1, pp. 1053, 1195)**

508. A. Four-fifths of diabetes mellitus cases occur as maturity onset, and most patients are obese at diagnosis. **(REF. 1, pp. 1053, 1195)**

509. C. An increased death rate at an early age is seen in both types, with incidence possibly improved on treatment. **(REF. 11, pp. 607, 617, 641)**

510. A. In type II, xanthomas are eruptive, appear when hyperlipemia is severe, and disappear when fat intake is reduced. **(REF. 11, pp. 607, 617, 641)**

511. B. Glucose intolerance is seen in many patients with familial type IV, but hypertriglyceridemia of this pattern occurs in diabetes. **(REF. 11, pp. 607, 617, 641)**

512. D. Increased chylomicrons are seen in type I and type V and have a high triglyceride content. **(REF. 11, pp. 607, 617, 641)**

513. B. In type IV, treatment includes reduction to ideal weight with low carbohydrate and no alcohol in the diet. Clofibrate and nicotinic acid are also tried. **(REF. 11, pp. 607, 617, 641)**

514. D. In addition to abnormal pigmentation, other manifestations of Addison's disease include anorexia, nausea, vomiting, lethargy, confusion, or psychosis. **(REF. 7, p. 281)**

198 / Diseases of Nutrition, Metabolism, and Endocrines

515. C. Cardiac changes in thyrotoxicosis may be auricular fibrillation and cardiomegaly. Other symptoms include palpitation, tachycardia, nervousness, sweating, and dyspnea. (**REF.** 7, pp. 186–189)

516. E. Thyroid biopsy may be useful in the diagnosis of all four conditions listed. Malignant lesions should not be biopsied by needle techniques but by open techniques to prevent seeding along the needle tract. (**REF.** 7, p. 171)

517. A. A pituitary tumor is not suspected by finding loss of hearing. Other signs of a pituitary tumor and symptoms include uncinate fits, rhinorrhea, papilledema, and hormone excess. (**REF.** 7, p. 105)

518. B. The release of vasopressin is controlled by hypertonicity of the blood perfusing the head and by volume receptors in the left atrium and vascular areas. Regulation of vasopressin is by osmotic stimuli and nonosmotic stimuli such as neural stimuli arising outside the hypothalamus. (**REF.** 7, p. 1032)

519. D. Nonfunctioning nodules of the thyroid should be considered possibly malignant. Unless metastasis or local extension becomes evident, no clinical means exists for establishing or excluding carcinoma. (**REF.** 7, p. 236)

520. D. The differential diagnosis of hypoglycemia includes tumor of the pancreatic beta cells. Classification of hypoglycemia includes spontaneous causes such as reactive or fasting hypoglycemia and pharmacologic or toxic causes. (**REF.** 7, p. 844)

521. C. Abnormalities in the tubular reabsorption of phosphate occur in hyperparathyroidism and in intrinsic renal disease with a BUN of 100 mg%. The renal handling of phosphate involves glomerular filtration, tubular reabsorption, and possibly tubular secretion. (**REF.** 7, p. 964)

522. E. In addition to all those listed, other signs and symp-

Diseases of Nutrition, Metabolism, and Endocrines / 199

toms of acromegaly include headache, visual impairment, weight gain, and hyperhidrosis. (REF. 7, p. 108)

523. B. Glucagon is secreted by the alpha cells of the pancreas and is effective in raising blood sugar levels. It also exerts a marked effect on carbohydrate, fat, and lipid metabolism and increases cyclic AMP in many tissues. (REF. 7, p. 749)

524. A. Hyperparathyroidism is not associated with a testicular carcinoma. Polyendocrine adenomatosis most frequently include the alpha cell tumors of the pancreas, leading to the Zollinger-Ellison syndrome. (REF. 7, p. 978)

525. B. Estrogen causes development of secondary sexual characteristics and thickening of the vaginal mucosa and cornification. The age of onset of pubertal changes and their rates of progression are subject to a number of variables. (REF. 7, p. 375)

526. D. Feminizing adrenocortical tumors are usually malignant. The commonest presenting sign or symptom is polymenorrhea or irregular bleeding alternating with amenorrhea. (REF. 7, p. 279)

527. B. Growth hormone produces hypertrophy with functional impairment in many tissues and may cause high glycogen content in the muscle. (REF. 7, p. 87)

528. A. Osteoporosis is not associated with vitamin D-resistant rickets. This is a familial disorder with an X-linked recessive pattern treated with pharmacologic doses of vitamin D. (REF. 11, p. 1541)

529. E. Diabetic ketosis is usually precipitated by all the factors cited. Marked hyperglycemia leads to marked glycosuria and an osmotic loss of water and electrolytes. (REF. 7, p. 806)

530. C. In gouty patients, serum urate levels are positively correlated with body weight and surface area. Obesity and hypertriglyceridemia may be associated diseases. (REF. 11, p. 916)

200 / Diseases of Nutrition, Metabolism, and Endocrines

531. E. In osteomalacia all four conditions may occur. In severe cases there is bowing of the long bones, inward deformity of the pelvic bones and wide osteoid borders on bone surfaces. **(REF. 1, p. 1337)**

532. A. Secondary hyperparathyroidism is not a complication of Paget's disease of the bone. The sacrum and pelvis are most frequently involved, followed closely by the tibia and femur. **(REF. 1, p. 1346)**

533. A. Vitamin D deficiency does not lead to decreased renal excretion of phosphorus. Many affected persons have no demonstrable abnormality except for hypophosphatemia. **(REF. 1, p. 1338)**

534. E. Ammonia levels in the blood are determined by all of the factors listed. The normal blood ammonia is less than 150 $\mu g\%$ but may rise as high as 500 $\mu g\%$ in liver disease. **(REF. 9, p. 684)**

535. C. In phenylketonuria a low-phenylalanine diet and a gluten-free diet to age 12 are required, with relentless attention to details of diet for a good outcome. **(REF. 9, p. 716)**

536. B. Cirrhosis of the liver and signs of basal ganglia disease are included in the triad of Wilson's disease. A brownish pigmented ring at the corneal margin is pathognomonic of the disease. **(REF. 1, p. 1126)**

537. D. Phenylketonuria is treated by a diet low in phenylalanine. Mental retardation becomes evident at 6 months of age unless diet is rigorously observed. **(REF. 1, p. 1101)**

538. B. Glucose phosphorylation is enhanced by insulin as is the activity of lipoprotein lipase in the presence of glucose. **(REF. 11, p. 96)**

539. A. Do not use salicylates in the treatment of thyroid storm even though there is severe hyperpyrexia, as salicylates increase free thyroid hormones and oxygen consumption. **(REF. 1, p. 1212)**

Diseases of Nutrition, Metabolism, and Endocrines / 201

540. E. The diagnosis is established by demonstration of cortisol levels less than 15 micrograms per decilitre, before and after an injection of ACTH. (**REF. 1, p. 1229**)

541. D. All of the causes listed may delay puberty, but the cause is almost always normal variation in growth pattern. (**REF. 1, p. 1247**)

542. C. Response to hormone therapy can be predicted in patients with metastases confined to bone, skin, lung, and nodes, and in those at least five years postmenopausal. (**REF. 1, p. 1284**)

543. B. A generally increased risk for breast cancer is associated with nulliparity, late first pregnancy, and especially a history of maternal breast cancer. (**REF. 1, p. 1283**)

544. E. Several patients with ovarian primaries have been described that have the systemic findings without demonstrated metastases. (**REF. 1, p. 1312**)

545. D. The diagnosis of primary hyperaldosteronism for practical purposes begins with the recognition that a patient has high blood pressure. (**REF. 7, pp. 277, 1066**)

546. C. Hyperaldosteronism is often associated with diabetic glucose tolerance curve. Hypokalemia as a diagnostic criterion is a convenience rather than a necessity. (**REF. 7, pp. 277, 1066**)

547. B. Adrenal surgery is the treatment. If adenomas are present they are removed. If no adenoma is found, one and a half adrenal glands are removed. (**REF. 7, p. 278**)

548. A. The pathology is a single, benign adenoma in the vast majority of cases. This syndrome may rarely be associated with diffuse hyperplasia, dependent on ACTH, angiotensin, or potassium. (**REF. 7, p. 277**)

549. D. Malignant hypertension with papilledema would rule out this syndrome. Primary aldosteronism may account for approximately 1% of the hypertensive population. **(REF. 7, p. 277)**

550. A. Diabetes mellitus is a syndrome consisting of hyperglycemia, large vessel disease, microvascular disease, and neuropathy. **(REF. 7, p. 758)**

551. B. An insulin tolerance test does not establish the diagnosis of diabetes mellitus. Blood analysis of glucose may rely on the glucose oxidase method, but the autoanalyzer uses the ferricyanide reagent. **(REF. 7, p. 782)**

552. E. Open-angle glaucoma is not revealed on eye examination. The earliest eye changes may be a functional disturbance of the blood vessels. **(REF. 7, p. 794)**

553. C. The patient is most likely to develop intercapillary glomerulosclerosis. There are three histological types of intercapillary glomerulosclerosis: nodular, diffuse, and exudative. **(REF. 7, p. 792)**

554. C. Pyoderma gangrenosum is not a cutaneous manifestation. Perineal pruritus in a diabetic is almost always associated with *Candida albicans.* **(REF. 7, p. 804)**

555. C. The diagnosis is hyperparathyroidism. Calcium deposits are seen in the periarticular areas of the fourth and fifth metacarpophalangeal, third proximal interphalangeal and fourth distal interphalangeal joints. There is slight soft tissue swelling, especially of the fourth and fifth metacarpophalangeal joints. Calcification in scleroderma is subcutaneous in location. In gout, if monosodium urate is deposited it could appear as a soft tissue mass. **(REF. 2, p. 1832)**

556. B. Autonomous adrenal tumors are ACTH insensitive and fail to demonstrate a brisk use in urinary 17-hydroxycorticoids. **(REF. 2, p. 1714)**

8. Diseases of the Musculoskeletal System

DIRECTIONS: Each of the questions or incomplete statements below is followed by five suggested answers or completions. Select the **one** that is **best** in each case.

557. Marfan's syndrome involves all of the following EXCEPT
    A. abnormalities of the eye
    B. marked obesity
    C. excessively long tubular bones
    D. kyphoscoliosis
    E. dissecting aneurysm

558. Systemic lupus erythematosus occurs most commonly in
    A. elderly women
    B. young men
    C. women of childbearing age
    D. elderly men
    E. children

559. The basic defect in the genetic mucopolysaccharidoses is
    A. insulin deficiency
    B. abnormal elastic tissue
    C. excess iron in tissue
    D. homocystinuria
    E. abnormal lysosomal enzymes

204 / Diseases of the Musculoskeletal System

560. Hepatitis in young women may be a manifestation of
  A. dermatomyositis
  B. systemic lupus erythematosus
  C. scleroderma
  D. thrombotic thrombocytopenic purpura
  E. periarteritis nodosa

561. Cardiac manifestations of polyarteritis nodosa may include (? except)
  A. hypertension
  B. coronary insufficiency
  C. pericarditis
  D. granulomatous myocarditis
  E. bicuspid aortic valve

562. Juvenile rheumatoid arthritis (Still's disease) is characterized by all of the following EXCEPT
  A. daily high fevers
  B. lymphadenopathy
  C. pleuritis
  D. cervical spondylitis
  E. tests for the rheumatoid factor that are usually positive

563. X-ray findings in degenerative joint disease (osteoarthritis) include all of the following EXCEPT
  A. narrowing of the joint space
  B. osteoporosis
  C. marginal lipping
  D. bony sclerosis
  E. irregularity of joint surfaces

564. Sjögren's syndrome (keratoconjunctivitis sicca) is associated with all of the following EXCEPT
  A. xerostomia
  B. inflammation in the salivary glands
  C. Aschoff nodules
  D. arthritis
  E. inflammation in the lacrimal glands

565. A diagnostically helpful ophthalmic finding in lupus erythematosus is
   A. cytoid bodies
   B. microaneurysm
   C. Argyll-Robertson pupil
   D. macular degeneration
   E. nystagmus

566. The most common portion of the gastrointestinal tract to become involved in scleroderma is the
   A. esophagus
   B. stomach
   C. duodenum
   D. ileum
   E. colon

567. Raynaud's phenomenon
   A. may lead to gangrene of the fingers
   B. is almost always due to scleroderma
   C. occurs when scleroderma is always well established
   D. causes fingers to turn red in cold water
   E. affects the sexes equally

568. Pseudogout can be distinguished from gout by means of
   A. positive birefringent crystals
   B. acute onset
   C. involvement of single joints
   D. involvement of large joints
   E. association with diabetes

569. Rheumatoid spondylitis is characterized by
   A. subcutaneous nodules
   B. low sedimentation rate
   C. positive sheep cell agglutination
   D. persistent activity for two or three years followed by spontaneous fusion of the spine
   E. affecting females predominantly

206 / Diseases of the Musculoskeletal System

570. Sjögren's syndrome involves all of the following EXCEPT
    A. xerophthalmia
    B. xerostomia
    C. lymphocytic infiltration of glands
    D. rheumatoid arthritis
    E. malignant lymphoma

571. The cardiac lesion commonly associated with rheumatoid spondylitis is
    A. aortic insufficiency
    B. aortic stenosis
    C. mitral insufficiency
    D. mitral stenosis
    E. multiple valve disease

572. Malignancy is classically associated with
    A. systemic lupus erythematosus
    B. scleroderma
    C. dermatomyositis
    D. polyarteritis
    E. Weber-Christian disease

573. Takayasu's syndrome is characterized by
    A. high pressure in the legs and low pressure in the arms
    B. low pressure in the legs and high pressure in the arms
    C. high-pitched diastolic murmur
    D. occurrence in old males
    E. hypertension

Diseases of the Musculoskeletal System / 207

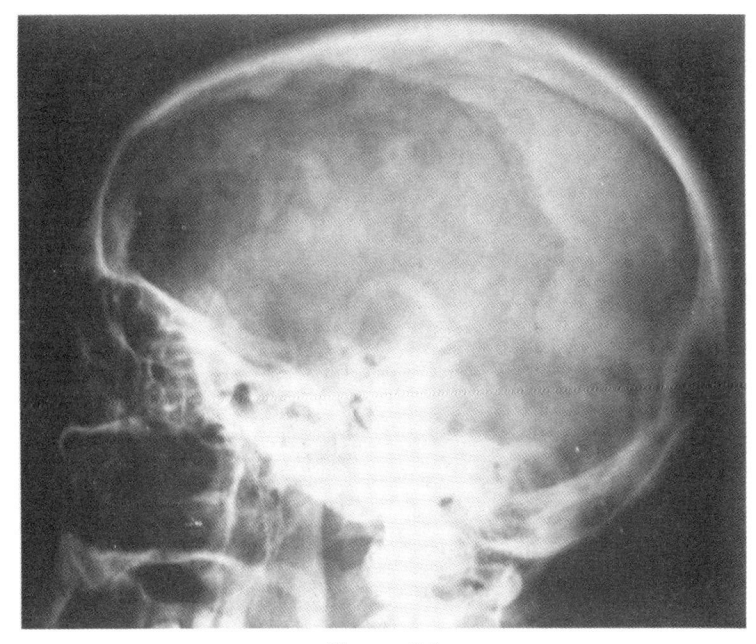

Figure 8.1

574. Figure 8.1 is the x-ray of a 40-year-old white male with symptoms of sinusitis and an incidental finding in the skull. What is your diagnosis?
   A. Normal variant
   B. Osteomyelitis
   C. Paget's disease
   D. Hemangioma
   E. Metastatic disease

208 / Diseases of the Musculoskeletal System

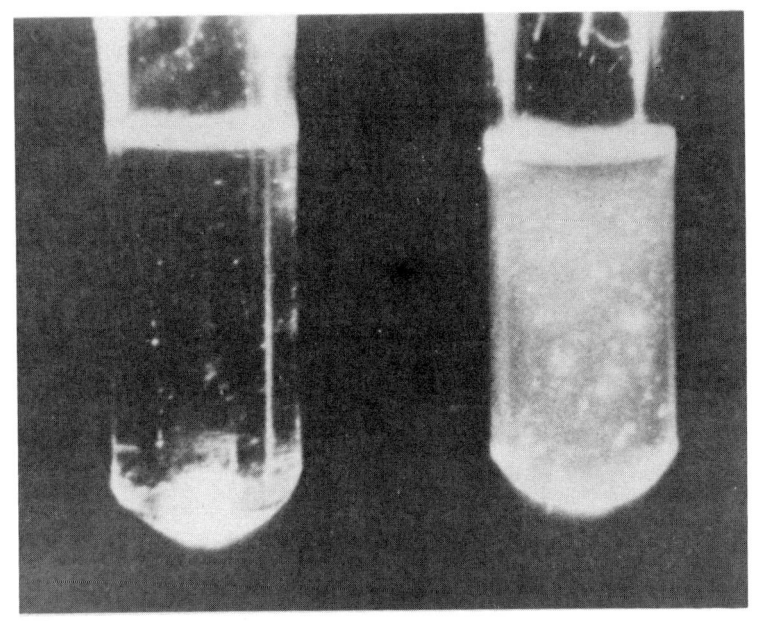

Figure 8.2

575. A mucin clot test is shown in Figure 8.2 with the normal control on the left and the patient's fluid on the right. What is the patient's most likely diagnosis?
    A. Degenerative joint disease
    B. Traumatic arthritis
    C. Systemic lupus
    D. Scleroderma
    E. Gout

576. Joint fluid aspiration is also analyzed for all of the following EXCEPT
    A. sodium content
    B. viscosity
    C. bacterial culture
    D. cytology
    E. inclusions

Diseases of the Musculoskeletal System / 209

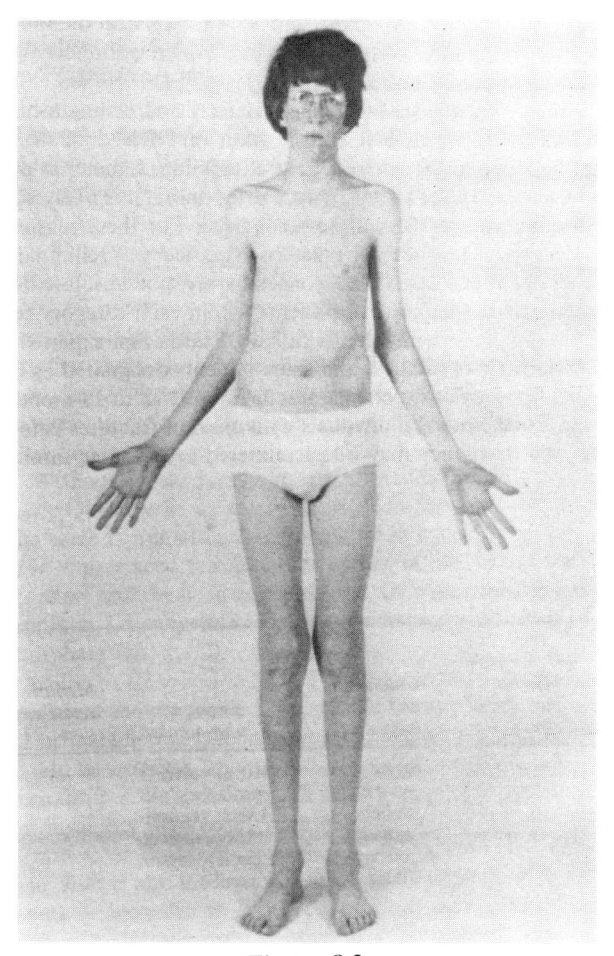

Figure 8.3

577. What is the usual cause of death in the condition pictured in Figure 8.3?
   A. Ruptured esophageal varices
   B. Berry aneurysm
   C. Aortic aneurysm
   D. Respiratory failure
   E. Sepsis

DIRECTIONS: Each set of lettered headings below is followed by a list of numbered words or phrases. For each numbered word or phrase select

- **A** if the item is associated with (A) *only*,
- **B** if the item is associated with (B) *only*,
- **C** if the item is associated with *both* (A) *and* (B),
- **D** if the item is associated with *neither* (A) *nor* (B).

    A. Juvenile rheumatoid arthritis
    B. Adult rheumatoid arthritis
    C. Both
    D. Neither

578. Predominantly in females

579. Severe systemic signs and symptoms

580. Involvement of the larger joints

581. Benefits by treatment with cortisone ointment

582. Test for rheumatoid factor usually positive

    A. Dermatomyositis
    B. Temporal arteritis
    C. Both
    D. Neither

583. Renal disease is common

584. Leukocytosis

585. Intensity of skin manifestations related to exposure to sun

586. Systemic manifestations

587. Optic atrophy

   A. Rheumatoid arthritis
   B. Osteoarthritis
   C. Both
   D. Neither

588. Pain relieved by rest, aggravated by use

589. Prolonged stiffness after rest

590. Cartilaginous and bony enlargement of the terminal interphalangeal joints of the fingers

591. Narrowing of joint spaces on x-ray

592. Lack of correlation between x-ray changes and symptoms

   A. Ankylosing spondylitis
   B. Reiter's syndrome
   C. Both
   D. Neither

593. Urethritis

594. HLA-B27

595. Single joint involvement

596. Aortic regurgitation

597. Rheumatoid factor

   A. Systemic lupus erythematosus
   B. Rheumatoid arthritis
   C. Both
   D. Neither

Diseases of the Musculoskeletal System

598. Preceding history of purpura in a patient with arthritis

599. Positive LE test

600. Rheumatoid factor

601. Subcutaneous nodules in about 10-20% of cases

602. Heberden's nodes

DIRECTIONS: For each of the questions or incomplete statements below, **one** or **more** of the answers or completions given is correct. Select
- A if only *1, 2 and 3* are correct,
- B if only *1 and 3* are correct,
- C if only *2 and 4* are correct,
- D if only *4* is correct,
- E if *all* are correct.

---

603. Leukopenia is a common finding in
    1. periarteritis nodosa
    2. scleroderma
    3. dermatomyositis
    4. systemic lupus erythematosus

604. Hypertrophic osteoarthropathy is associated with
    1. periosteal inflammation
    2. rheumatoid factor
    3. new bone formation
    4. aortic stenosis

605. The skin manifestations of polyarteritis include
    1. subcutaneous nodules
    2. bullous dermatitis
    3. livedo racemosa
    4. hyperpigmentation

Diseases of the Musculoskeletal System / 213

606. The arthritis accompanying ulcerative colitis is usually associated with
1. coincident regional enteritis
2. progressive crippling course
3. symmetrical small joint involvement
4. asymmetric involvement of the knees and ankles

607. Psoriatic arthritis is characterized by
1. distal interphalangeal joint involvement
2. association with sacroiliitis
3. nail lesions
4. "pencil-in-cup" deformity

608. Ankylosing spondylitis is characterized by
1. chronicity
2. involvement of the sacroiliac joints
3. possible fusion of the entire spine
4. highest frequency in older women

609. In temporal arteritis
1. the sexes are equally represented
2. the major age group affected is 50 to 80 years
3. the mortality rate is less than 2%
4. there is a visual complication in over 50% of cases

610. Characteristic features of Wegener's granulomatosis include
1. nodular pulmonary lesions
2. intractable rhinitis and sinusitis
3. terminal uremia
4. congestive heart failure

611. The rheumatoid factor
1. is positive in almost 100% of "classical" rheumatoid arthritis
2. is only seen in rheumatoid arthritis
3. has a molecular weight of about 160,000
4. is positive in 10% to 20% of juvenile rheumatoid arthritis

Directions Summarized				
A	B	C	D	E
1,2,3	1,3	2,4	4	All are
only	only	only	only	correct

612. Rheumatic fever
1. is causally related to the group B Streptococcus
2. is related to the beta-hemolytic Streptococcus
3. is not seen in epidemics in the family unit
4. usually shows a rise in antistreptolysin titer in the acute phase

613. The Ehlers-Danlos syndrome is characterized by
1. hyperelastic skin
2. mental retardation
3. habitual dislocation of joints
4. increased incidence of skin carcinoma

614. Important findings in the diagnosis of rheumatic fever include
1. erythema marginatum
2. chorea
3. polyarthritis
4. subcutaneous nodules

615. Which of the following are synovial fluid characteristics in traumatic arthritis?
1. Bloody
2. Poor mucin clot
3. Small fibrin clot
4. 5,000 to 50,000 WBC per mm^3

616. In dermatomyositis the course of muscle necrosis can be followed by repeated
1. sedimentation rates
2. serum transaminase enzymes
3. electromyography
4. muscle biopsies

Diseases of the Musculoskeletal System / 215

DIRECTIONS: This section consists of situations, each followed by a series of questions. Study each situation, and select the **one** best answer to each question following it.

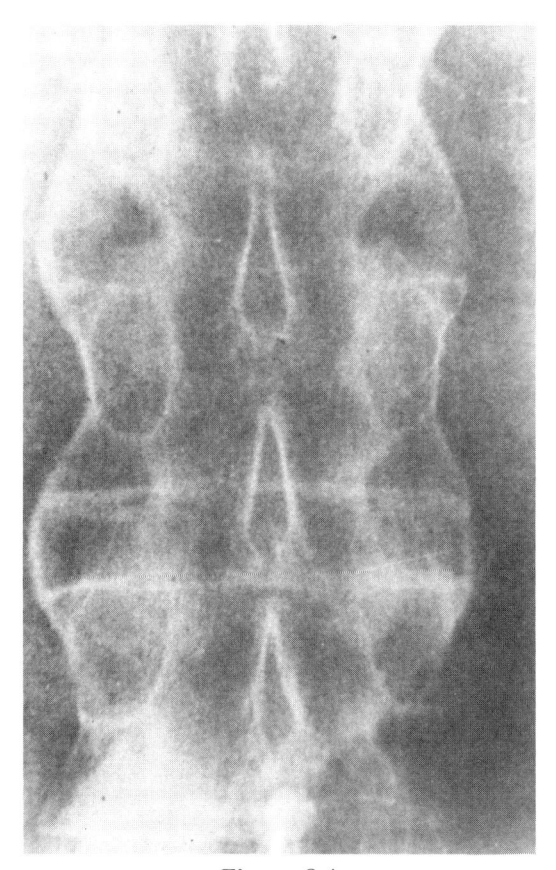

Figure 8.4

CASE 1 (Questions 617-620): A 22-year-old man has a history of low back pain and stiffness. After several months of mild symptoms, he notes more severe stiffness at night and hip pain. On physical examination there is paravertebral muscle tenderness and limited flexion of the lumbar spine. A diastolic murmur is heard. Figure 8.4 shows an x-ray of the lumbar spine.

216 / Diseases of the Musculoskeletal System

617. What is the most likely diagnosis?
    A. Reiter's syndrome
    B. Marfan's syndrome
    C. Ankylosing spondylitis
    D. Rheumatoid arthritis
    E. Pseudogout

618. What is the diastolic murmur likely to be?
    A. Mitral stenosis
    B. Tricuspid stenosis
    C. Aortic insufficiency
    D. Pulmonic insufficiency
    E. Tetralogy of Fallot

619. What is the most likely extra-articular manifestation of this disease?
    A. Colitis
    B. Iridocyclitis
    C. Psoriasis
    D. Urethritis
    E. Cardiac conduction disturbances

620. All of the following are recommended for therapy of this conditions EXCEPT
    A. indomethacin
    B. phenylbutazone
    C. exercise programs
    D. sleep without a pillow
    E. radiotherapy

8. Diseases of the Musculoskeletal System Answers and Comments

557. B. In Marfan's syndrome, inheritance is autosomal dominant, and the aortic lesion is a cystic medial necrosis with loss of elastic tissue. The syndrome does not include marked obesity. **(REF. 1, p. 1138)**

558. C. SLE is more frequent in blacks than whites and rare among Asians; it is five to ten times more common in women of childbearing age. **(REF. 1, p. 1852)**

559. E. Each syndrome in the genetic mucopolysaccharidoses is caused by a mutation-produced deficiency in the activity of a lysosomal enzyme. **(REF. 2, pp. 922-923)**

560. B. Lupoid hepatitis is a condition of young women with progressive active hepatitis, but SLE may lead to transient fatty infiltration. **(REF. 1, p. 790)**

561. E. The first four conditions listed may be cardiac manifestations. Heart failure is responsible for or contributes to death in one sixth to one-half of polyarteritis nodosa cases. **(REF. 1, p. 1866)**

562. E. In Still's disease, tests for the rheumatoid factor are not always positive. In about 25% of patients, especially when less than 6 years old, prominent systemic symptoms occur. **(REF. 2, pp. 1875, 1879)**

563. B. Osteoporosis is not a finding in osteoarthritis. Early pathologic changes occur in the joint cartilage; subsequently, new bone formation develops. **(REF. 2, pp. 1894, 1896)**

564. C. Sjögren's syndrome is not associated with Aschoff nodules. The lack of secretions may also involve the entire respiratory tract, vagina, and skin. **(REF. 1, p. 1861)**

218 / Diseases of the Musculoskeletal System

565. A. Cytoid bodies are a diagnostically helpful ophthalmic finding. Other systems involved in LE include skin, cardiopulmonary, neurologic, and lymph node. **(REF. 2, p. 355)**

566. A. Esophageal symptoms are present in more than 50% of patients. **(REF. 2, p. 1370)**

567. A. Raynaud's phenomenon may lead to gangrene of the fingers. The soft tissue of the fingertips is lost, and the bone of the terminal phalanges may be resorbed. **(REF. 2, p. 1897)**

568. A. Pseudogout is distinguishable from gout by positive birefringent crystals. Calcium pyrophosphate crystals are short, blunt rhomboids, and urate crystals are needle-shaped with negative birefringence. **(REF. 2, p. 1888)**

569. D. Rheumatoid spondylitis is characterized by persistent activity for two or three years followed by spontaneous fusion of the spine. Cervical spine disease is common, but the lower spine is relatively spared. **(REF. 2, p. 1880)**

570. E. Development of massive lymphadenopathy, splenomegaly, and leukopenia suggests malignant lymphoma but is considered hyperplasia. **(REF. 2, p. 1879)**

571. A. Aortic insufficiency is commonly associated with rheumatoid spondylitis. Cystic medial necrosis with loss of elastic tissue is the underlying pathology. **(REF. 2, pp. 1149, 1876)**

572. C. Most tumors associated with dermatomyositis have been bronchogenic carcinomas, but many others have occurred. **(REF. 2, p. 2053)**

573. A. High pressure in the legs and low pressure in the arms characterize Takayasu's syndrome. Clinical manifestations include easy fatigability of the arms and atrophy of the soft tissues of the face. **(REF. 2, p. 1178)**

574. C. There is a rarefied area involving the frontal and parietal bones. This is an early stage of Paget's disease where calvarial thickening and foci or radiopacity are not present within the radiolucent area. At this stage of the disease, a cross-section through the margin of the lesion reveals a compact inner and outer table in the normal portion, while the diploe widens and extends to the outer and inner surfaces of the calvarium without a change in the calvarial thickness in the lesion. **(REF. 2, p. 1861)**

575. E. When acetic acid is added, a good ropy clot forms in normal joint fluid, but a poor clot forms in severe inflammatory arthritis, including gout and rheumatoid arthritis. **(REF. 1, p. 1841)**

576. A. Other analyses may include Gram stain, white count and differential, color, crystals, proteins, and rheumatoid factor. **(REF. 1, p. 1840)**

577. C. The patient has Marfan's syndrome. Aortic involvement occurs in about 80%, with degenerative changes predominating. **(REF. 1, p. 1138)**

578. C. Females are affected with both forms three times more commonly than males. **(REF. 2, pp. 1872, 1876)**

579. A. Patients with juvenile rheumatoid arthritis may have high fever, rash lymphadenopathy, splenomegaly, and hepatomegaly. **(REF. 2, p. 1879)**

580. A. One-third of patients with juvenile rheumatoid arthritis have monoarticular arthritis, usually in the knee or ankle. **(REF. 2, p. 1879)**

581. D. Salicylates are the mainstay of treatment in both forms, along with rest and physiotherapy. **(REF. 2, p. 1879)**

582. B. Only 10% to 20% of juvenile rheumatoids have positive rheumatoid factor. **(REF. 2, p. 1879)**

583. D. Autopsy has shown renal arteritis, but clinical disease is rare in either condition. **(REF. 1, pp. 1871, 1872)**

584. C. In both conditions, leukocytosis is moderate and is largely due to increased neutrophils. **(REF.** 1, pp. 1871, 1872)

585. A. In dermatomyositis, skin rashes can mimic erythema nodosum, eczema, or exfoliative dermatitis. **(REF.** 1, pp. 1871, 1872)

586. C. Systemic manifestations in both conditions include fever, weakness, anemia, and leukocytosis. **(REF.** 1, pp. 1871, 1872)

587. B. In temporal arteritis, sudden onset of blindness may occur in one or both eyes from ophthalmic or vertebral artery disease. **(REF.** 1, pp. 1871, 1872)

588. C. In both conditions, judicious rest and a mixture of exercise and physiotherapy are used to prevent deformity. **(REF.** 1, pp. 1845, 1882)

589. A. In rheumatoid arthritis, morning stiffness is an almost invariable feature, and severity varies with the extent of the disease. **(REF.** 1, pp. 1845, 1882)

590. B. Heberden's nodes are bony protuberances at the dorsal margins of distal interphalangeal joints, which appear in osteoarthritis. **(REF.** 1, pp. 1845, 1882)

591. C. Aside from joint narrowing, osteophyte formation is seen in degenerative joint disease, but radiolucent subchondral cysts are seen in both. **(REF.** 1, pp. 1845, 1882)

592. B. In osteoarthritis, deformities characterizing Heberden's nodes may be marked but these are not associated with pain or inflammation. **(REF.** 1, pp. 1845, 1882)

593. B. In Reiter's syndrome, gonococcal urethritis may usher in the nonspecific urethritis, so that a smear and a culture should be done. **(REF.** 1, pp. 1878, 1879)

594. A. HLA-B27 has a striking incidence in ankylosing

Diseases of the Musculoskeletal System / 221

spondylitis and may indicate genetic factors in etiology. **(REF. 1, pp. 1878, 1879)**

595. B. The distribution of the arthritis in Reiter's syndrome tends to be asymmetric, and single or multiple joints may be involved. **(REF. 1, pp. 1878, 1879)**

596. C. The pathogenesis of aortic regurgitation is similar in both diseases, with medial necrosis of the aortic root and dilatation of the aortic ring. **(REF. 1, pp. 1878, 1879)**

597. D. Tests for the rheumatoid factor are negative in both diseases, and rheumatoid nodules are not seen in either. **(REF. 1, pp. 1878, 1879)**

598. A. Idiopathic thrombocytopenic purpura often remits only to advance to SLE years later. **(REF. 2, pp. 355, 1872)**

599. C. In both conditions, the LE cell test may indicate the presence of antinuclear antibodies and is inhibited by anti-complementary factors. **(REF. 2, pp. 355, 1872)**

600. C. The rheumatoid factor is found in both conditions. It consists of heterogeneous antibodies, IgM, IgG, and IgA, specific for IgG. **(REF. 2, pp. 355, 1872)**

601. B. In rheumatoid arthritis, subcutaneous nodules are most commonly located over the extensor surface of elbows but also over the fingers, the back of head, and the sacrum. **(REF. 2, pp. 355, 1872)**

602. D. Heberden's nodes are seen in degenerative joint diseases over the distal interphalangeal joints. **(REF. 2, pp. 355, 1872)**

603. D. Leukopenia occurs in about one-half of the SLE patients, and the differential count is usually normal. **(REF. 1, p. 1852)**

604. B. Periosteal inflammation and new bone formation are

222 / Diseases of the Musculoskeletal System

associated with hypertrophic osteoarthropathy. Round cell infiltration and edema develop in the periosteum, synovial membrane, and joint capsule. **(REF. 2, p. 1900)**

605. B. Acute manifestations include polymorphic exanthemas that are purpuric, erythematous, and multiform. **(REF. 1, p. 1866)**

606. D. The arthritis accompanying ulcerative colitis is usually associated with asymmetric involvement of the knees and ankles. Also reported in ulcerative colitis is a more common association with erythema nodosum and uveitis than is found in other types of arthritis. **(REF. 1, p. 703)**

607. E. Psoriatic arthritis is characterized by all four conditions. Resorption of the distal end of the bone produces the "pencil," which projects into a cuplike erosion in the adjacent joint surface. **(REF. 2, p. 1884)**

608. A. Ankylosing spondylitis is characterized by chronicity, involvement of the sacroiliac joints, and possible fusion of the entire spine. Recent studies have demonstrated a striking association between HLA-B27 and ankylosing spondylitis. **(REF. 1, p. 1878)**

609. C. In temporal arteritis, the major age group affected is 50 to 80 years and there is a visual complication in over 50% of cases. Large and medium-sized arteries are involved, with inflammation and giant cells but no necrosis. **(REF. 2, p. 1940)**

610. A. In Wegener's granulomatosis, arteries, arterioles, venules, and capillaries are involved with necrotizing inflammation. Congestive heart failure is not a characteristic feature. **(REF. 2, pp. 352, 935)**

611. D. The rheumatoid factor is positive in 10% to 20% of juvenile rheumatoid arthritis cases. One-third of patients have monoarticular arthritis, most often in a knee or an ankle. **(REF. 2, p. 1879)**

612. C. Rheumatic fever is related to the beta-hemolytic

Diseases of the Musculoskeletal System / 223

Streptococcus. The antistreptolysin O titer will rise in 80% of streptococcal group A infections. **(REF. 2, p. 1090)**

613. B. In the Ehlers-Danlos syndrome, skin hyperextensibility, fragility, and bruisability are marked, and this condition may create difficulties at operation. Habitual dislocation of joints is also a characteristic of this syndrome. **(REF. 2, p. 530)**

614. E. All four of the conditions listed are important in the diagnosis. The joint pains are characteristically fleeting and migratory, with no permanent joint deformities. **(REF. 2, p. 1090)**

615. B. In traumatic arthritis, swellings, ecchymoses, muscular spasms, and tenderness tend to be present, but fractures must be excluded. Synovial fluid is bloody and has a small fibrin clot. **(REF. 2, p. 1871)**

616. C. The course of muscle necrosis can be followed by repeated serum transaminase enzymes and by repeated muscle biopsies. The creatine excretion in the urine is moderately elevated in most cases and creatinine excretion is low. **(REF. 2, p. 2054)**

617. C. The disease is 30 times more prevalent among the relatives of patients than the general population. There is a striking association with the histocompatibility antigen HLA-B_{27}. **(REF. 1, p. 1878)**

618. C. The frequency of aortic insufficiency has been about 4%. Other cardiac valve anomalies are not increased in incidence. **(REF. 1, p. 1879)**

619. B. Iridocyclitis occurs in about one-quarter of patients. Cardiac conduction disturbances occur in about 10%. **(REF. 1, p. 1879)**

620. E. Radiotherapy was formerly used to reduce pain and inflammation but was associated with a 10-fold incidence of leukemia. **(REF. 1, p. 1879)**

9. Diseases of the Nervous System

DIRECTIONS: Each of the questions or incomplete statements below is followed by five suggested answers or completions. Select the **one** that is **best** in each case.

621. Early signs of cord compression in extramedullary tumors are all of the following EXCEPT
    A. spastic weakness of the muscles below the level of the lesion
    B. loss of heat and cold sensation below the level of the lesion
    C. impairment of cutaneous and proprioceptive sensation below the level of the lesion
    D. increase in the reflexes
    E. impairment of bladder control

622. Alzheimer's disease (presenile dementia) is associated with
    A. atrophy of the frontal and temporal poles
    B. atrophy of the entire frontal and temporal lobes
    C. cranial nerve palsies
    D. transient episodes of hemiplegia
    E. hemianesthesia

Diseases of the Nervous System / 225

623. Chronic progressive chorea (Huntington's) is characterized by all of the following EXCEPT
    A. hereditary disorder
    B. childhood onset
    C. mental deterioration
    D. atrophy of the cortex
    E. enlargement of the ventricles on pneumoencephalogram

624. The incubation period of rabies from animal bite to signs of disease is
    A. shortest when the wound is on the leg
    B. shortest when the wound is on the face
    C. prolonged by tetracycline but not prevented
    D. two years
    E. one week

625. Migraine headaches may be associated with all of the following focal neurologic signs EXCEPT
    A. diplopia
    B. dysphasia
    C. paresthesia
    D. weakness
    E. seizure

626. A history of progressive loss of hearing, tinnitus, and ataxia is suspicious of
    A. Meniere's disease
    B. acoustic neuroma
    C. otitis media
    D. increased intracranial pressure
    E. cerebellar hemangioblastoma

627. An elderly patient with onset of malaise, weight loss, increased ESR, and temporal arteritis probably has
    A. glioblastoma multiforme
    B. multiple sclerosis
    C. systemic lupus erythematosus
    D. polymyalgia rheumatica
    E. meningitis

226 / Diseases of the Nervous System

628. A patient with amyotrophic lateral sclerosis develops a loss of emotional control with outbursts of laughing or crying that are inappropriate. The patient has probably developed
  A. an agitated depression
  B. schizophrenia
  C. brain stem infarction
  D. a posterior fossa tumor
  E. pseudobulbar palsy

629. The diagnosis in an infant with convulsions, chorioretinitis, and x-ray evidence of calcification of the brain is most likely to be
  A. Tay-Sachs disease
  B. hydrocephalus
  C. kernicterus
  D. toxoplasmosis
  E. congenital neurosyphilis

630. Occlusion of the right posterior cerebral artery is most likely to cause
  A. homonymous hemianopia
  B. total blindness
  C. sudden death
  D. infarction of the right brain stem
  E. a right-sided hemiplegia

631. In amyotrophic lateral sclerosis, one finds
  A. a long history of remissions and exacerbations
  B. sensory loss in the distribution of peripheral nerves
  C. focal seizures
  D. signs of ventral horn and lateral column involvement
  E. cogwheel rigidity

632. Transient episodes of vertigo, slurred speech, diplopia, and paresthesias suggest
    A. basilar artery insufficiency
    B. anterior communicating artery aneurysm
    C. hypertensive encephalopathy
    D. psuedobulbar palsy
    E. occlusion of the middle cerebral artery

633. Hemorrhage into the extradural space is generally due to
    A. anterior fossa bleeding
    B. middle meningeal artery tear
    C. dural sinus tear
    D. bilateral bleeding
    E. brain tumor

634. A right homonymous hemianopia is due to a lesion of the
    A. right optic nerve
    B. chiasm
    C. right optic radiations
    D. right occipital lobe
    E. left optic radiations

635. Neonatal meningitis is frequently due to
    A. a genitourinary infection in the mother
    B. neonatal otitis media
    C. a skull fracture
    D. septicemia at birth
    E. tuberculosis

636. Cafe-au-lait spots are seen in association with
    A. atrophy of the proximal musculature
    B. optic atrophy
    C. multiple subcutaneous nodules
    D. congenital nystagmus
    E. mental retardation

228 / Diseases of the Nervous System

637. A lesion of the oculomotor nerve can result in
    A. paralysis of the lateral gaze
    B. ptosis of the eyelid
    C. widening of the palpebral fissure
    D. inability to turn the eye downward and outward
    E. deviation of the eye inward

638. Injury to the ulnar nerve results in
    A. atrophy of the muscles of the thenar eminence
    B. wrist drop
    C. inability to oppose the thumb
    D. sensory loss of the palmar surface of the thumb, index, and middle fingers
    E. impaired adduction and abduction of the fingers

639. In a patient with subacute combined degeneration of the spinal cord
    A. either folic acid or vitamin B_{12} can be used in treatment
    B. vibration sensation in the lower extremities is usually unimpaired
    C. the pathologic changes in the nervous system involve the gray matter to a much greater extent than the white matter
    D. the neurologic manifestations may precede the blood changes
    E. the cerebrospinal fluid is diagnostic

640. A 63-year-old man suddenly becomes acutely ill and has a fever of 102.4°F. There is pain in the eye and the orbits are painful to pressure. There is edema and chemosis of the conjunctivas and eyelids. The bulbs are proptosed. There is diplopia and ptosis, and the pupils are slow in reacting. The most likely diagnosis is
    A. cavernous sinus thrombosis
    B. chorioretinitis
    C. subarachnoid hemorrhage
    D. brain abscess
    E. none of these

641. The syndrome of familial periodic paralysis may be associated with all of the following EXCEPT
A. hyperkalemia
B. hypokalemia
C. normokalemia
D. hypercalcemia
E. epinephrine sensitivity

642. A 20-year-old girl presents with a history of rapid loss of vision in one eye. Examination reveals pain on movement of the eyeball. The pupillary reactions are normal as is the appearance of the fundi. Perimetry shows a large central scotoma. The most likely diagnosis is
A. optic atrophy
B. papilledema
C. retrobulbar neuritis
D. amblyopia ex anopsia
E. hysteria

643. A tumor of the central nervous system which has a tendency to metastasize to other areas of the cerebrum and spinal cord is
A. an oligodendroglioma
B. a meningioma
C. an ependymoma
D. a medulloblastoma
E. a craniopharyngioma

644. The combination of polyneuritis and confusion, disorientation, loss of memory, and tendency to confabulate is most likely due to
A. pernicious anemia
B. alcoholism
C. cerebrovascular disease of the carotid system
D. Charcot-Marie-Tooth disease
E. dermatomyositis

230 / Diseases of the Nervous System

645. A 67-year-old man has episodes lasting up to 5 minutes, which consist of numbness of the left side of his body with impaired vision in his right eye. The most likely diagnosis is
   A. posterior cerebral artery insufficiency
   B. parietal lobe neoplasm
   C. parasagittal meningioma
   D. AV malformation
   E. internal carotid artery insufficiency

646. Signs and symptoms of involvement of the peripheral nerves in the form of pains, paresthesias, motor weakness, and reflex loss develop in a fairly large percentage of patients with
   A. heart disease
   B. dermatomyositis
   C. hypothyroidism
   D. diabetes mellitus
   E. adrenal insufficiency

647. A subdural hematoma
   A. is practically always of venous origin
   B. is rarely seen in infancy
   C. is due to injury to the middle meningeal artery
   D. is always chronic
   E. does not usually occur in the absence of trauma

648. The most common type of intracranial tumor is
   A. a meningioma
   B. a pituitary adenoma
   C. a metastatic tumor
   D. an angioma
   E. a glioma

649. Intervertebral disc rupture with signs of cord compression is best treated by
   A. strict bed rest on a firm surface
   B. potent muscle relaxants
   C. immediate surgery
   D. observation, including myelograms
   E. leg traction

650. The major cause of aneurysms in the subarachnoid space is
  A. trauma
  B. tumor
  C. syphilis
  D. congenital weakness
  E. septic emboli

651. An acoustic neuroma is most likely to lead to a palsy of the
  A. fourth cranial nerve
  B. sixth cranial nerve
  C. eighth cranial nerve
  D. tenth cranial nerve
  E. eleventh cranial nerve

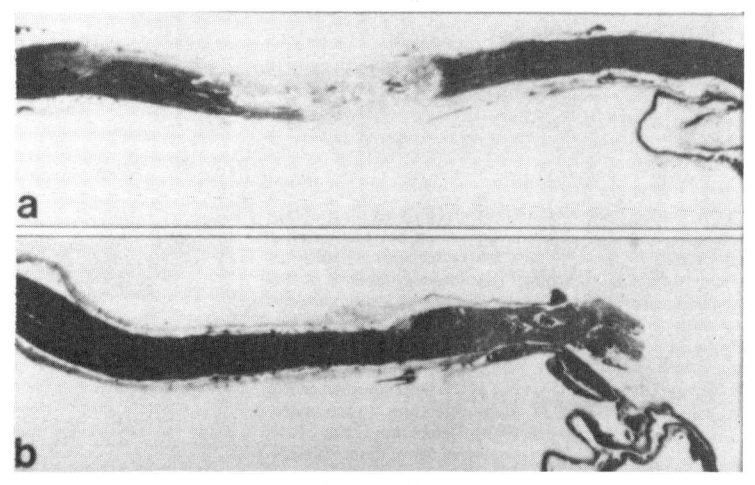

Figure 9.1

652. Figure 9.1,a shows a plaque of demyelination in the optic nerve as compared to a normal sample in Figure 9.1,b. What is the most likely cause of this phenomenon?
  A. Diabetic microvascular disease
  B. Arteriosclerosis
  C. Trauma
  D. Multiple sclerosis
  E. Jakob-Creutzfeldt disease

232 / Diseases of the Nervous System

653. Which of the following is the LEAST common presenting symptom in the disease illustrated above?
    A. Leg weakness
    B. Paresthesias
    C. Visual loss
    D. Sphincter impairment
    E. Incoordination

DIRECTIONS: For each of the questions or incomplete statements below, **one** or **more** of the answers or completions given is correct. Select
    A   if only *1, 2 and 3* are correct,
    B   if only *1 and 3* are correct,
    C   if only *2 and 4* are correct,
    D   if only *4* is correct,
    E   if *all* are correct.

---

654. Cryptococcosis
    1. may simulate tuberculous meningitis
    2. may produce nodules indistinguishable from Hodgkin's disease
    3. is usually fatal
    4. occurs only in leukemia

655. In tuberous sclerosis which of the following may be found?
    1. Facial nevi
    2. Mental retardation
    3. Renal tumors
    4. Convulsions

656. Muscular wasting and/or atrophy can occur in
    1. syringomyelia
    2. Cushing's syndrome
    3. amyotrophic lateral sclerosis
    4. myasthenia gravis

657. In familial periodic paralysis the
     1. serum potassium level is usually low
     2. injection of glucose and insulin can produce an attack
     3. condition is hereditary
     4. attacks grow progressively worse with advancing age

658. Tremors are seen in
     1. hyperthyroidism
     2. acute alcoholism
     3. hepatic coma
     4. myxedema

659. The pathologic changes in Friedreich's ataxia are found in the
     1. basal ganglia
     2. cerebral cortex
     3. peripheral autonomic nerves
     4. spinal cord tracts

660. The bones of the skull may be involved in
     1. xanthomatosis
     2. multiple myeloma
     3. osteitis deformans
     4. osteitis fibrosa cystica

661. In hepatolenticular degeneration (Wilson's disease), there is usually
     1. a reduction of copper excretion in the urine
     2. a reduction of the serum ceruloplasmin content
     3. no renal involvement
     4. a peculiar greenish brown pigmentation of the cornea

Directions Summarized

A	B	C	D	E
1,2,3 only	1,3 only	2,4 only	4 only	All are correct

662. Ophthalmoplegia may be found in which of the following?
    1. Migraine
    2. Ophthalmic zoster
    3. Myasthenia gravis
    4. Paralysis agitans

663. Involvement of the optic chiasm with defects in the visual fields can occur in
    1. a pituitary adenoma
    2. a craniopharyngioma
    3. an aneurysm of the internal carotid artery
    4. a falx meningioma

664. Fasciculations can be found in which of the following conditions?
    1. Myotonic muscular dystrophy
    2. Amyotonia congenita
    3. Tabes dorsalis
    4. Amyotrophic lateral sclerosis

665. The cardinal features of Parkinson's disease (paralysis agitans) include
    1. constant fine tremor
    2. muscle atrophy
    3. pupillary constriction
    4. akinesia

Diseases of the Nervous System / 235

666. Hydrocephalus may result from which of the following?
1. Aqueductal stenosis
2. Absence of the foramina of Luschka
3. Adhesions in the meningeal space in the basal cisterns
4. Agenesis of the corpus callosum

667. Demyelinization within the central nervous system may be a feature in which of the following conditions?
1. Vascular lesions
2. Infectious processes
3. Nutritional deficiencies
4. Post-vaccinal

668. Seizures following head injury
1. are inevitable
2. may indicate a brain abscess
3. usually occur immediately
4. are more often generalized than focal

669. Syringomyelia is characterized by
1. gliosis and cavitation
2. atrophy and fibrillation of muscles
3. muscular wasting
4. segmental loss of pain and temperature sensation

236 / Diseases of the Nervous System

DIRECTIONS: This section consists of situations, each followed by a series of questions. Study each situation, and select the **one** best answer to each question following it.

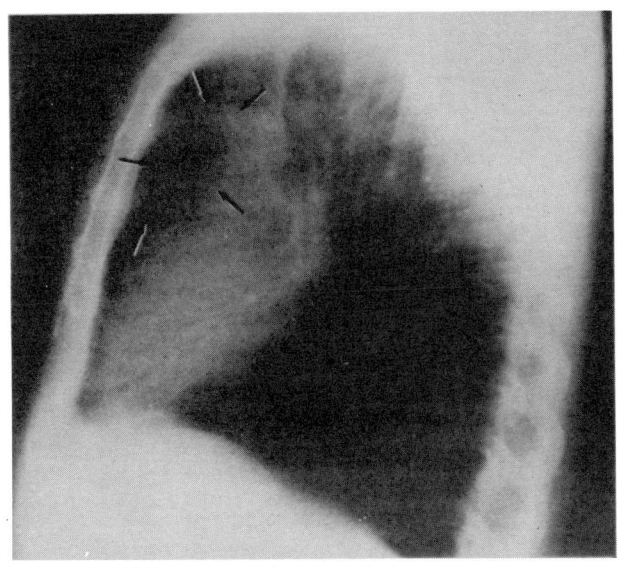

Figure 9.2

CASE 1 (Questions 670-672): A 37-year-old woman complains of drooping eyelids at the end of the day. Further history reveals difficulty in chewing food and some weakness in climbing stairs. On examination there is weakness of eyelids, masticatory muscles, and thigh flexors. There is no sensory abnormality and reflexes are normal. The chest x-ray is shown in Figure 9.2.

670. What does the chest x-ray show?
   A. Bronchogenic carcinoma
   B. Hodgkin's disease
   C. Teratoma
   D. Thyroid tumor with retrosternal extension
   E. Thymoma

671. What is the cause of the patient's symptoms?
    A. Hypercalcemia
    B. Myasthenia gravis
    C. Multiple sclerosis
    D. Thyroid storm
    E. Meningeal lymphoma

672. All of the following treatments may be used in this patient EXCEPT
    A. adrenergic drugs
    B. surgery
    C. plasmapheresis
    D. cholinergic drugs
    E. steroids

238 / Diseases of the Nervous System

9. Diseases of the Nervous System Answers and Comments

621. B. Early signs do not include loss of heat and cold sensation below the level of the lesion. Benign tumors of the spinal cord are characterized by a slowly progressive course extending over several years. **(REF. 6, p. 304)**

622. B. Alzheimer's disease is associated with atrophy of the entire frontal and temporal lobes. Microscopically, there is diffuse loss of cells in all layers, secondary gliosis, and neurofibrillar degeneration. **(REF. 6, pp. 484-489)**

623. B. The most common onset is the appearance of abnormal movements, but it may include psychotic episodes or frank mental deterioration. Huntington's chorea is not characterized by onset in childhood. **(REF. 6, pp. 493-498)**

624. B. The incubation period is shortest when the wound is on the face. Onset of disease is signalled by pain or numbness in the region of the bite, followed by apathy, drowsiness, headache, and anorexia. **(REF. 6, p. 80)**

625. E. Migraine headaches are not associated with seizure. Since migraine is a functional disorder, it is rare for the symptoms to occur in the same location at every attack. **(REF. 6, p. 830)**

626. B. By the time the acoustic neuroma is recognized clinically, it is mainly intracranial and of a large size. **(REF. 6, p. 249)**

627. D. In polymyalgia rheumatica there is no weakness, the serum enzymes are normal, and there are no muscle changes on biopsy or EMG. **(REF. 6, pp. 628-629)**

628. E. The patient has probably developed pseudobulbar palsy. The weakness of the muscles is usually symmetrical and in the terminal stages of disease is generalized. **(REF. 6, pp. 190, 555)**

629. D. Toxoplasmosis is the most likely diagnosis. The infection has a predilection for the central nervous system and the eye and produces encephalitis in utero. **(REF. 6, pp. 122-124)**

630. A. Occlusion of the right posterior cerebral artery is most likely to cause homonymous hemianopia. This artery conveys blood to the inferior and medial portion of the posterior temporal and occipital lobes and to the optic thalamus. **(REF. 6, p. 188)**

631. D. Signs of ventral horn and lateral column involvement are found in myotrophic lateral sclerosis. The most severe changes are in the region of the corticospinal tract as well as in the anterior roots and the peripheral nerves. **(REF. 6, pp. 549-558)**

632. A. Basilar artery insufficiency is suggested by the transient episodes. The basilar artery is formed by the two vertebral arteries and supplies the pons, the midbrain, and the cerebellum. **(REF. 6, p. 190)**

633. B. Hemorrhage into the extradural space is generally due to middle meningeal artery tear. The size of the clot increases until the ruptured vessel is occluded by clot formation. Bilateral bleeding is extremely rare. **(REF. 6, p. 329)**

634. E. The hemaniopia is due to a lesion of the left optic radiations. The posterior cerebral artery arises from the basilar artery but is sometimes a branch of the internal carotid. **(REF. 6, p. 188)**

635. A. Neonatal meningitis is often due to a genitourinary infection in the mother. The pathology, symptomatology, and clinical course of patients with acute purulent meningitis are similar regardless of the organism. **(REF. 6, p. 1)**

240 / Diseases of the Nervous System

636. C. Cafe-au-lait spots are seen in association with multiple subcutaneous nodules. Neurofibromatosis is an inherited disorder with multiple tumors of the spinal or cranial nerves, tumors of the skin, and cutaneous pigmentation. (**REF.** 6, pp. 314-319)

637. B. The lesion can result in ptosis of the eyelid. There is also loss of the ability to open the eye, and the eyeball is deviated outward and slightly downward. (**REF.** 6, p. 378)

638. E. Injury to the ulnar nerve results in impaired adduction and abduction of the fingers. The fibers arise from the eighth cervical and the first thoracic segments. The ulnar is a mixed nerve with sensory supply to the medial hand. (**REF.** 6, pp. 399-400)

639. D. The neurologic manifestations may precede the blood changes. The pathologic changes in the nervous system are essentially degenerative and affect the white matter more than the grey. (**REF.** 6, pp. 710-714)

640. A. Cavernous sinus thrombosis is usually secondary to suppurative processes in the orbit, the nasal sinuses, or the upper half of the face. (**REF.** 6, pp. 42-43)

641. D. The familial periodic paralysis syndrome is usually associated with low potassium, but normal or high levels may occur. It is characterized by recurrent attacks of weakness or paralysis of the somatic musculature, with loss of the deep tendon reflexes and may be aggravated by epinephrine. (**REF.** 6, pp. 606-607)

642. C. In the vast majority of cases, retrobulbar neuritis occurs as an episode in a demyelinating disease such as multiple sclerosis. (**REF.** 6, p. 785)

643. D. Medulloblastomas constitute about 10% of gliomas and are predominantly found in the cerebellum. (**REF.** 6, p. 258)

644. B. The combination is most likely due to alcoholism. Pain in the legs and paresthesias are quickly followed by weakness of the legs, foot drop, and ataxia. **(REF. 6, pp. 742–744)**

645. E. Internal carotid artery insufficiency is the most likely diagnosis. Abnormalities are found in the extracranial arteries in more than one-half of the patients with symptomatic cerebral infarction. **(REF. 6, p. 186)**

646. D. These signs and symptoms develop in a fairly large percentage of patients with diabetes mellitus. Loss of proprioceptive sensation together with absent reflexes superficially resembles tabes dorsalis. **(REF. 6, p. 762)**

647. A. A subdural hematoma is practically always of venous origin. It is almost always secondary to a minor or severe injury to the head but may occur in blood dyscrasias or cachexia in the absence of trauma. **(REF. 6, pp. 334–335)**

648. E. A glioma is the most common type of intracranial tumor. Next in order of frequency is meningioma, pituitary adenoma, and acoustic neuroma. **(REF. 6, p. 214)**

649. C. Immediate surgery is the best treatment. When cord compression is absent, more conservative measures are used, such as rest, a brace, traction, or neck extension. **(REF. 6, p. 367)**

650. D. Intracranial aneurysms are found in approximately 4% of all autopsies performed on adults. Their major cause is congenital weakness of the vessel wall. **(REF. 6, p. 200)**

651. C. An acoustic neuroma is most likely to lead to a palsy of the eighth cranial nerve. Deafness, headache, ataxia, tinnitus, and diplopia are seen, as well as facial paresthesias. **(REF. 6, p. 249)**

652. D. Visual loss in multiple sclerosis varies from slight blurring to no light perception. Other eye symptoms include diplopia and pain. (**REF.** 1, p. 211)

653. D. Weakness, especially of the legs, is the major presenting symptom of multiple sclerosis. Both sphincter impairment and vertigo occur at presentation in about 6% of the cases. (**REF.** 1, p. 2110)

654. A. Some success with amphotericin B has been reported in cryptococcosis, with treatment continued until the CSF is normal or toxicity occurs. The infection does not occur only in leukemia. (**REF.** 6, pp. 21–24)

655. E. All of the conditions listed may be found in tuberous sclerosis. Congenital tumors, and malformations in the nervous system, skin, and elsewhere develop in early life. (**REF.** 6, pp. 453–460)

656. E. Muscular wasting and atrophy can occur in all four conditions cited. Weakness and atrophy in myasthenia gravis are due to a defect in transmission at the myoneural junction. (**REF.** 6, pp. 224–227, 565, 549, 600)

657. A. Although hypokalemia is most common, potassium may also be normal or high in familial periodic paralysis. Attacks do not grow progressively worse with advancing age. (**REF.** 6, pp. 607–609)

658. A. Tremors are seen in hyperthyroidism, acute alcoholism, and hepatic coma. In hyperthyroidism, neurologic symptoms include tremors of the hands, exophthalmos, lid lag, stare, and muscle weakness. (**REF.** 6, pp. 691, 728, 742)

659. D. The pathologic changes are found in the spinal cord tracts. Degeneration is seen in the posterior funiculi, the lateral corticospinal tract, and the spinocerebellar tracts. (**REF.** 6, p. 536)

660. E. In addition to all of the conditions listed, the skull may also be affected by osteomas, hemangiomas, and metastatic carcinomas. (**REF.** 6, pp. 235–237)

Diseases of the Nervous System / 243

661. C. In Wilson's disease, there is usually a reduction of the serum ceruloplasmin content and a peculiar greenish brown pigmentation of the cornea. Signs and symptoms of injury to the basal ganglia are accompanied by cirrhosis of the liver. **(REF. 6, pp. 678-683)**

662. B. Ophthalmoplegia may be found in migraine and myasthenia gravis. Weakness of the facial and levator palpebrae muscles produces a characteristic expressionless facies with drooping of the eyelids. **(REF. 6, pp. 600, 835)**

663. A. Involvement can occur in the first three conditions listed. Adenomas of the pituitary gland constitute approximately 15% of intracranial tumors, with the chromophobic type most common. **(REF. 6, pp. 263, 274-276, 377)**

664. D. In approximately two-thirds of the patients with amyotrophic lateral sclerosis, the initial symptom of the disease is weakness and wasting of the extremities. **(REF. 6, p. 555)**

665. D. The cardinal features of Parkinson's disease include akinesia. The chief signs are masklike facies, dysarthria, alternating tremor, stooped posture, abnormal gait, and rigidity. **(REF. 6, pp. 509-515)**

666. A. Adults may develop hydrocephalus as a result of occlusion of CSF pathways by tumors in the third ventricle, brain stem, or posterior fossa. Hydrocephalus does not result from agenesis of the corpus callosum. **(REF. 6, p. 428)**

667. E. Demyelinization may be a feature in all of the conditions cited. Myelin is a complex protein-lipid carbohydrate structure, which forms part of the cell membrane of the oligodendroglia. **(REF. 6, p. 767)**

668. C. Seizures following head injury may indicate a brain abscess and are more often generalized than focal. In the majority of cases, seizures do not develop until several months after the injury, 6 to 18 months being the most common interval. **(REF. 6, pp. 321, 347)**

669. E. In addition to all of the characteristics listed, syringomyelia is frequently associated with other congenital defects, such as spina bifida, hydrocephalus, cranial malformations, or clubfeet. **(REF. 6, pp. 564–569)**

670. E. The thymus tissue is often abnormal, with encapsulated tumors occurring in about 15% of cases. Almost all thymomas occur in patients over 30. **(REF. 1, p. 2181)**

671. B. The most common presenting symptoms relate to weakness of eye muscles causing ptosis or diplopia. Difficulty in chewing, dysarthria, and dysphagia are also common. **(REF. 1, p. 2181)**

672. A. Cholinergic drugs are largely inhibitors of cholinesterase. Prednisone may improve as many as 80% of patients. Thymectomy helps patients with no thymoma, but thymoma patients don't do as well. Plasmapheresis benefits most patients but needs to be repeated at intervals. **(REF. 1, p. 2183)**

10. Clinical Pharmacology

DIRECTIONS: Each of the questions or incomplete statements below is followed by five suggested answers or completions. Select the **one** that is **best** in each case.

673. The administration of hydrochlorothiazide may cause
    A. increased serum potassium
    B. metabolic acidosis
    C. potassium loss and alkalosis
    D. respiratory alkalosis
    E. sodium retention

674. Corticosteroids are most helpful in the management of diffuse lung disease due to
    A. chemical injuries
    B. occupational dust
    C. chronic organizing pneumonia
    D. hemosiderosis
    E. scleroderma

675. Antidiuretic hormone acts by
    A. increasing the permeability of the proximal renal tubule to water
    B. increasing the permeability of the distal renal tubule to water
    C. decreasing the glomerular filtration rate
    D. increasing sodium excretion
    E. causing active reabsorption of water from the loop of Henle

246 / Clinical Pharmacology

676. Methimazole (Tapazole) interferes with thyroid function mainly by
    A. inhibition of iodine uptake
    B. inhibition of thyroidal organic-binding and coupling reactions
    C. immunologic means
    D. destruction of thyroid cells
    E. the same mechanism as perchlorate

677. A lupuslike picture may follow the administration of
    A. diphenylhydantoin
    B. estrogens
    C. hydralazine
    D. ergotamine
    E. Mustargen

678. Ampicillin (alpha-aminobenzyl penicillin) is
    A. not effective orally
    B. not inactivated by penicillinase
    C. acid stable
    D. not effective against coliform organisms
    E. not allergenic

679. Barbiturate overdosage is treated by all of the following EXCEPT
    A. forced diuresis
    B. gastric lavage
    C. cathartics
    D. positive pressure respiration
    E. dialysis

680. Untoward side effects of phenothiazines include all of the following EXCEPT
    A. sensory loss
    B. parkinsonismlike symptoms
    C. dystonic movements
    D. hypotensive episodes
    E. convulsive seizures

Clinical Pharmacology / 247

681. Quinidine produces a decrease in all of the following electrophysiologic properties of the myocardium EXCEPT
    A. the effective refractory period
    B. automaticity
    C. membrane responsiveness
    D. the conduction velocity
    E. excitability

682. Which of the following drugs requires a major adjustment in dosage in the presence of renal disase?
    A. Tetracycline
    B. Methicillin
    C. Erythromycin
    D. Chloramphenicol
    E. Ampicillin

683. Bronchodilators include all of the following EXCEPT
    A. ephedrine
    B. aminophylline
    C. isoproterenol hydrochloride
    D. potassium iodide
    E. epinephrine

684. Which of the following is the drug of choice for treatment of chronic myelogenous leukemia?
    A. Triethylenemelamine (TEM)
    B. Urethan (ethyl carbamate)
    C. Chlorambucil (Leukeran)
    D. Busulfan (Myleran)
    E. Amethopterin (Methotrexate)

685. All of the following stimulate gastric secretion EXCEPT
    A. ethyl alcohol
    B. acetylcholine
    C. reserpine
    D. caffeine
    E. fats

248 / Clinical Pharmacology

686. Xerostomia or dryness of the mouth may result from all of the following EXCEPT
    A. infection of salivary glands
    B. atropine
    C. gingivitis
    D. antihistamines
    E. Sjögren's syndrome

687. Thiocyanate and perchlorate are examples of agents that
    A. inhibit thyroglobulin release
    B. increase BMR
    C. inhibit iodide transport
    D. inhibit thyroid organic binding
    E. increase thyroxin synthesis

688. The principal toxic reaction to isoniazid is
    A. rash
    B. fever
    C. agranulocytosis
    D. peripheral neuritis
    E. hives

689. Estimation of barbiturates in the blood
    A. may be diagnostic in a patient in a coma of unknown etiology
    B. revealing a level of 2 mg% in a comatose patient is usually due to poisoning with long-acting barbiturates
    C. revealing a level of 12 mg% in a comatose patient is usually due to poisoning with long-acting barbiturates
    D. is quite reliable with the methods available
    E. correlates with salicylate levels

690. Propranolol may be used in the presence of
    A. asthma
    B. hypertrophic subaortic stenosis
    C. sinus bradycardia
    D. ether
    E. cardiogenic shock

691. Folic acid is best absorbed
    A. as a monoglutamate
    B. in the distal ileum
    C. with alcohol
    D. in pernicious anemia
    E. in the presence of abnormal gut bacteria

692. Vitamin B_{12} absorption is characteristically
    A. totally dependent on the intrinsic factor
    B. best in the duodenum
    C. improved in folic acid deficiency
    D. best in the distal ileum
    E. prevented by antiparietal cell antibodies

693. The thiocarbamides (Tapazole) exert their antithyroid effect by
    A. inhibiting the action of proteases on thyroglobulin
    B. competing with the iodide in the iodide-trapping system
    C. inhibiting the iodination of tyrosine
    D. making the thyroid refractory to thyrotropin
    E. inhibiting several important steps, which include the conversion of iodide to iodine in the thyroid

694. All of the following are properties of insulin EXCEPT
    A. increase in the permeability of some cells to glucose
    B. stimulation of RNA formation
    C. movement of potassium into cells
    D. promotion of fat synthesis
    E. effectiveness in the absence of intact cells

695. Folic acid, when administered to patients with pernicious anemia, is capable of producing all of the following EXCEPT
    A. a hematopoietic response
    B. relief of the neurologic manifestations
    C. relief of the glossitis
    D. an exacerbation of the neurologic signs
    E. a further lowering of the serum B_{12} level

250 / Clinical Pharmacology

696. Metyrapone (SU-4885) acts by blocking
    A. 11-hydroxylation
    B. 21-hydroxylation
    C. 17-hydroxylation
    D. the release of cortisol
    E. pituitary suppression

697. An overdose of lysergic acid diethylamide (LSD) is most likely to be associated with
    A. pupillary dilatation
    B. pupillary constriction
    C. bradycardia
    D. blindness
    E. deafness

698. Which of the following drugs reach effective levels in the cerebrospinal fluid?
    A. Kanamycin
    B. Vancomycin
    C. Polymyxin
    D. Oxytetracycline
    E. Penicillin V

699. Calcium absorption from the intestine is dependent on
    A. vitamin D only
    B. parathyroid hormone only
    C. the vitamin A level in blood
    D. vitamin D and parathyroid hormone
    E. alkaline phosphatase

700. The major side effects in patients receiving tetracycline have been
    A. neutropenia
    B. allergic reactions
    C. hepatitis
    D. gastrointestinal symptoms
    E. polyuria

701. The purpose of digitalis in established atrial fibrillation is to
   A. restore sinus rhythm
   B. slow the atrial rate
   C. slow the ventricular rate
   D. treat congestive heart failure
   E. depress the vagus nerve

DIRECTIONS: Each group of questions below consists of a list of lettered headings followed by a list of numbered words, phrases, or statements. For **each** numbered word, phrase or statement, select the **one** lettered heading that is most closely associated with it. Each lettered heading may be selected once, more than once, or not at all.

   A. Combines with cytochromes and catalase to block hydrogen and electron transport, thus producing tissue asphyxia
   B. Methemoglobinemia
   C. Vertigo, hyperventilation, tinnitus, and deafness
   D. Bone marrow depression
   E. Acute hepatic insufficiency

702. Chlorinated hydrocarbons

703. Salicylates

704. Cyanide

705. Benzene

706. Aniline dyes

DIRECTIONS: The set of lettered headings below is followed by a list of numbered words or phrases. For each numbered word or phrase select

    A if the item is associated with (A) *only*,
    B if the item is associated with (B) *only*,
    C if the item is associated with *both* (A) *and* (B),
    D if the item is associated with *neither* (A) *nor* (B).

    A. Alcohol
    B. Opiates
    C. Both
    D. Neither

707. High incidence of addiction

708. Pancreatitis

709. Nutritional value

710. Amblyopia

711. Methadone treatment

    A. Verapamil
    B. Bretylium
    C. Both
    D. Neither

712. Interferes with the movement of calcium

713. Following administration there is a transient increase in heart rate and blood pressure

714. Permits conversion of refractory ventricular fibrillation when DC cardioversion has failed

715. May be the treatment of choice in acute paroxysmal AV junctional tachycardias

Clinical Pharmacology / 253

DIRECTIONS: For each of the questions or incomplete statements below, **one** or **more** of the answers or completions given is correct. Select
 A if only *1, 2 and 3* are correct,
 B if only *1 and 3* are correct,
 C if only *2 and 4* are correct,
 D if only *4* is correct,
 E if *all* are correct.

716. In quinidine-induced thrombocytopenic purpura
  1. there is a relation of dose to degree of thrombocytopenia
  2. there is a more common incidence in males
  3. thrombocytopenia lasts three weeks following cessation of the drug
  4. antibodies may be demonstrated for as long as six months

717. The treatment of choice for acute adrenal insufficiency is
  1. prednisolone
  2. 6-methylprednisolone
  3. dexamethasone
  4. cortisol phosphate

718. Nitroglycerin has the effect of
  1. increasing cardiac venous return
  2. diminishing cardiac output
  3. constricting peripheral veins and capillaries
  4. dilating coronary arteries

719. Which are the peak effects of the various insulins?
  1. Regular insulin at 8 hours
  2. Regular insulin at 2 hours
  3. Protamine insulin at 2 hours
  4. NPH insulin at 12 hours

254 / Clinical Pharmacology

Directions Summarized				
A	B	C	D	E
1,2,3 only	1,3 only	2,4 only	4 only	All are correct

720. True hepatotoxic drugs, as compared to those inducing a hypersensitivity reaction, would include
   1. chlorpromazine
   2. chloroform
   3. sulfonamides
   4. carbon tetrachloride

721. Which of the following are iatrogenic effects of the administration of anti-inflammatory steroids?
   1. Psychosis
   2. Thrombophlebitis
   3. Peptic ulcer
   4. Fever

722. Allopurinol effectively
   1. blocks uric acid production
   2. blocks excretion of uric acid by renal tubular mechanisms
   3. inhibits xanthine oxidase
   4. diminishes inflammation of acute gouty arthritis

723. Heparin therapy
   1. is active by mouth
   2. affects hepatic synthesis of factors
   3. is monitored by prothrombin time
   4. may be neutralized by protamine

724. Patients should receive preoperative steroids if they have had significant treatment with these drugs within
   1. one month of surgery
   2. three months of surgery
   3. six months of surgery
   4. three years of surgery

725. The best treatment of the adrenogenital syndrome in females consists of
    1. cortisol suppression of ACTH
    2. administration of 17-ketosteroids
    3. administration of dexamethasone in the hypertensive variety
    4. castration

726. Excessive use of furosemide may lead to
    1. acidosis
    2. dehydration
    3. hyperkalemia
    4. alkalosis

727. Antibiotics that distribute well to cerebrospinal fluid include
    1. streptomycin
    2. sulfonamides
    3. tetracycline
    4. chloramphenicol

728. Methotrexate is metabolized predominantly by
    1. pulmonary excretion
    2. hepatic conjugation
    3. alkylation
    4. renal excretion

729. Cimetidine is beneficial in the treatment of peptic ulcer because it
    1. blocks histamine–H_1 receptors
    2. is well absorbed in the stomach
    3. can be taken once daily
    4. almost totally abolishes basal acid secretion

730. Which of the following correctly describes furosemide?
    1. No effect in the presence of hypoalbuminemia
    2. Chemically related to sulfonamides
    3. Affects only the proximal tubules
    4. May cause "contraction alkalosis"

Directions Summarized				
A	B	C	D	E
1,2,3 only	1,3 only	2,4 only	4 only	All are correct

731. Which of the following is true in reference to anthracyclines?
    1. Major site of metabolism is in tumor tissue
    2. Acute cardiac arrhythmias may occur
    3. DNA but not RNA is affected, after administration in vivo
    4. Extravasation leads to severe local reaction

732. Prophylaxis for deep vein thrombosis in patients undergoing surgery may consist of
    1. minidose heparin
    2. phenylbutazone
    3. postoperative warfarin
    4. acetaminophen

10. Clinical Pharmacology
Answers and Comments

673. C. Administration of hydrochlorothiazide may cause potassium loss and alkalosis. The mechanism is most probably increased delivery of sodium to sites where secretion of hydrogen and potassium occur. **(REF. 8, p. 1711)**

674. A. Corticosteroids are most helpful in diffuse lung disease due to chemical injuries. Steroids are also helpful in lung disease due to hypersensitivity pneumonia, sarcoidosis, histiocytosis X, and desquamative pneumonia. **(REF. 8, p. 1479)**

675. B. No direct effect of vasopressin on sodium excretion has been observed in man, but water retention may secondarily induce sodium excretion. **(REF. 8, p. 916)**

676. B. Methimazol interferes with thyroid function mainly by inhibition of thyroidal organic-binding and coupling reactions. In contrast to other agents such as perchlorate, the action of thionamides is not prevented by large doses of iodide. **(REF. 8, p. 1411)**

677. C. A lupuslike picture may follow administration of hydralazine. Renal disease and central nervous system involvement are very unusual in drug-induced disease. **(REF. 8, p. 799)**

678. C. Polar side chains added to penicillin molecules made these compounds acid stable and therefore improved absorption. **(REF. 8, p. 1143)**

679. C. Barbiturate overdosage is not treated with cathartics. Dialysis is reserved for profound intoxication due to long-acting barbiturates after trial or other methods. **(REF. 8, p. 359)**

680. A. Sensory loss is not a side effect of phenothiazines. Parkinsonismlike symptoms disappear when phenothiazine is withdrawn. Dystonic movements involve the mouth, tongue, and shoulder girdle. (**REF.** 8, p. 408)

681. A. The refractory period increase accounts for the effect on tachycardias. Similar effects are seen with procainamide. (**REF.** 8, p. 770)

682. A. Tetracycline requires a major adjustment in dosage in the presence of renal disease. An injection may accentuate azotemia by its catabolic effect in increasing nitrogen turnover. (**REF.** 8, p. 1184)

683. D. Potassium iodide is not a bronchodilator. It assists in the liquefaction of sputum, as does glyceryl guaiacolate. (**REF.** 8, p. 592)

684. D. Busulfan is the drug of choice. It is an alkylating agent given by mouth, with onset of effect 10 to 14 days after the start of therapy. (**REF.** 8, p. 1268)

685. E. Fats release cholecystokinin, which inhibits gastric secretion. (**REF.** 8, p. 94)

686. C. Xerostomia does not result from gingivitis. Radiation of salivary glands may cause permanent dryness secondary to gland atrophy. (**REF.** 8, p. 126)

687. C. Because of their toxicity, neither drug is widely used in treatment, but both are effective in inhibiting iodide transport. (**REF.** 8, p. 1412)

688. D. Peripheral neuritis and optic neuritis are minimized by treatment with pyridoxine. (**REF.** 8, p. 1202)

689. A. Estimation of barbiturates in the blood may be diagnostic in a patient in a coma of unknown etiology. The production of barbiturates by drug companies greatly exceeds the amount needed for therapeutic purposes, so that addiction and overdose are common problems. (**REF.** 8, p. 549)

Clinical Pharmacology / 259

690. B. Propranolol may be used in the presence of hypertropic subaortic stenosis. Beta-adrenergic blockade will exacerbate allergies, bradycardias, and myocardial dysfunction. **(REF. 8, p. 188)**

691. A. Folic acid is present in food as polyglutamates and is deconjugated to a monoglutamate by intestinal enzymes. **(REF. 8, p. 1340)**

692. D. Vitamin B_{12} absorption is best in the distal ileum. Receptors for the intrinsic factor are present in the distal ileum, but mass action absorption also occurs with large doses. **(REF. 8, p. 1337)**

693. E. The inhibiting action is directed at the coupling of iodotyrosines, the iodination of MIT to form DIT and the formation of MIT. **(REF. 8, p. 1411)**

694. E. Insulin is not effective in the absence of intact cells. Insulin is synthesized as proinsulin with 86 amino acids and is then split into two chains connected by sulfur bridges. **(REF. 8, p. 1497)**

695. B. Folic acid administered to patients with pernicious anemia does not produce relief of the neurologic manifestations. Folate and B_{12} metabolism are intertwined, so that B_{12} is low in folate deficiency and red cell folate is low in B_{12} deficiency. **(REF. 8, p. 1340)**

696. A. Metyrapone acts by blocking 11-hydroxylation. The final step in cortisol biosynthesis is catalyzed by 11-beta-hydroxylase. **(REF. 8, p. 1492)**

697. A. Sympathomimetic effects such as pupillary dilatation, piloerection, hyperthermia, and tachycardia are common in an overdosage of LSD. **(REF. 8, p. 564)**

698. E. Penicillin reaches effective levels in the CSF. Drugs such as the sulfonamides, tetracycline, streptomycin, and erythromycin reach high levels in the presence of meningeal inflammation. (REF. 8, p. 1135)

699. D. Calcium absorption from the intestine is dependent on vitamin D and parathyroid hormone. A major target tissue for vitamin D is the intestinal mucosa, where it increases the transport of calcium. (REF. 8, p. 1538)

700. D. Gastrointestinal symptoms are the major side effects of tetracycline. Stomatitis, glossitis, and diarrhea are seen and may be related to superinfections. (REF. 8, p. 1181)

701. C. The purpose is to slow the ventricular rate. Overdigitalization may interfere with electric shock or quinidine therapy. (REF. 8, p. 729)

702. E. In chronically poisoned patients, cerebellar symptoms and evidence of liver damage may develop, especially with hexachlorobenzene. (REF. 8, p. 1655)

703. C. Salicylates are associated with vertigo, hyperventilation, tinnitus, and deafness. Excretion of salicylates is renal, and in the presence of normal renal function about 50% will be excreted in 24 hours. (REF. 8, p. 695)

704. A. Inhalation of hydrogen cyanide may cause death within a minute; oral doses act more slowly, requiring several minutes to hours. Cyanide combines with cytochromes and catalase to produce tissue asphyxia. (REF. 8, p. 1651)

705. D. Benzene is associated with bone marrow depression. Benzene is present to some extent in most gasolines, and poisoning may result from ingestion or from vapors. (REF. 8, p. 1647)

706. B. Headaches, dizziness, hypotension, convulsions, and coma may occur in methemoglobinemia, and jaundice and anemia may be late sequelae. (REF. 8, p. 702)

707. C. Both alcohol and opiates have a high incidence of addiction. Children may exhibit an increased susceptibility to opiates, so that relatively small doses may prove toxic. **(REF. 8, pp. 376, 494)**

708. A. Alcohol is associated with pancreatitis. The mildest forms may go unnoticed unless revealed by a transient elevation of the serum amylase level. **(REF. 8, pp. 376, 494)**

709. D. Opiates have no nutritional value and contrary to prevailing opinion, beers and liquors have too low a vitamin B content to be of nutritional value. **(REF. 8, pp. 376, 494)**

710. C. Amblyopia is associated with both. In heroin addicts it is probably due to the toxic effects of quinine in the mixtures. **(REF. 8, pp. 376, 494)**

711. B. Methadone is used to control the addiction to heroin, but it requires daily administration and the patient is dependent on the methadone. **(REF. 8, pp. 376, 494)**

712. A. Verapamil appears to exert its effect by interfering with movement of calcium through the so-called "slow channel." **(REF. 1, p. 286)**

713. B. Bretylium initially causes a release of catecholamines followed by sympathetic blockade. **(REF. 1, p. 286)**

714. B. Bretylium prolongs the refractoriness of tissues in the His-Purkinje system as well as the ventricles. **(REF. 1, p. 286)**

715. A. The slow channel calcium blockade has considerable importance in the region of the sinus node and the AV node. **(REF. 1, p. 286)**

716. D. Antibodies may be demonstrated for as long as six months. Thrombocytopenia develops within 12 hours of ingesting quinidine and the severity is not dose-related. **(REF. 8, p. 1056)**

717. D. Cortisol phosphate is the treatment of choice. Rapid intravenous infusion of physiologic saline may also be lifesaving. **(REF.** 8, p. 1482)

718. C. The benefit of nitroglycerin is probably due to diminution in cardiac output and work of the heart and to dilation of coronary arteries. **(REF.** 8, p. 825)

719. C. Semilente peaks at 3 to 6 hours, lente at 6 to 10 hours, PZI at 10 to 16 hours, regular insulin at 2 hours, and NPH at 12 hours. **(REF.** 8, p. 1497)

720. C. Chloroform and carbon tetrachloride are true hepatotoxic drugs that have a predictable dose-related toxicity and a short latent period. **(REF.** 8, pp. 291, 1645)

721. A. Fever is not an iatrogenic effect of anti-inflammatory steroids. Occasionally, muscle-wasting progresses to the point where it is objectively apparent. **(REF.** 8, p. 1482)

722. B. Allopurinol effectively blocks uric acid production and inhibits xanthine oxidase. Allopurinol is indicated in patients with a history of uric acid calculi of the urinary tract. **(REF.** 8, p. 720)

723. D. Heparin rebound refers to the reappearance of heparin in the circulation after apparent neutralization with protamine. **(REF.** 8, p. 1348)

724. A. Patients should receive preoperative steroids if they have had significant steroid treatment within six months of surgery. **(REF.** 8, p. 1482)

725. B. The best treatment is cortisol suppression of ACTH and dexamethasone in the hypertensive variety. Failure to suppress with dexamethasone is justification for a search for adrenal tumor. **(REF.** 8, p. 1482)

726. C. In addition to dehydration, hypokalemia, hypochloremia, and alkalosis also result from excessive use of furosemide. **(REF.** 8, p. 903)

Clinical Pharmacology / 263

727. C. Antibiotics that distribute well include sulfonamides and chloramphenicol. Some drugs such as penicillin, tetracycline, or streptomycin distribute in the CSF only during meningeal infection. **(REF. 8, pp. 1109, 1192)**

728. D. Methotrexate levels must be continuously measured following high-dose therapy until renal excretion is complete. **(REF. 8, p. 1274)**

729. D. Cimetidine blocks histamine–H_2 receptors, is well absorbed in the small intestine, but is taken four times daily or twice daily in long-acting form. **(REF. 1, p. 647)**

730. C. Furosemide is effective despite gross electrolyte disturbances or hypoalbuminemia. Excretion of large volumes of bicarbonate-poor urine leads to alkalosis. **(REF. 1, p. 153)**

731. C. Anthracyclines include daunorubicin and doxorubicin. The major site of metabolism is the liver, and the mechanism of action includes inhibition of DNA-dependent RNA metabolism. **(REF. 1, p. 1043)**

732. B. Minidose heparin may be given two hours preoperatively and continued as 5000 units subcutaneously every twelve hours. **(REF. 1, p. 329)**

11. Diseases of the Skin

DIRECTIONS: Each of the questions or incomplete statements below is followed by five suggested answers or completions. Select the **one** that is **best** in each case.

733. Koebner's phenomenon (lesions at the site of trauma) is typically seen in
    A. psoriasis
    B. eczema
    C. hypersensitivity reactions
    D. hyperkeratosis
    E. toxic erythemas

734. Kaposi's sarcoma often manifests as
    A. multiple blue dermal plaques
    B. melanotic nodules
    C. eczema
    D. maculopapular rash
    E. serum-filled bullae

735. Psoriasis may present all of the following clinical manifestations EXCEPT
    A. sharp demarcation of lesions at the hairline
    B. progression of lesions unless therapy is applied
    C. drop-shaped lesions
    D. extensive large plaques
    E. pitting of the nails

Diseases of the Skin / 265

736. Which of the following does NOT occur in dermatomyositis?
    A. Discoloration of the upper eyelids
    B. Loss of pigmentation
    C. Sensitivity to light
    D. Calcification of subcutaneous tissue
    E. Dermatitis herpetiformis

737. The best treatment of atopic dermatitis includes
    A. psychoanalysis
    B. warm clothing
    C. dry environment
    D. a change of environment
    E. vigorous exercise

738. Keratoacanthoma is best characterized by
    A. slow growth
    B. slow involution
    C. usual occurrence on the trunk
    D. a malignant potential
    E. a dark-brown color

739. Of the following, the area LEAST likely to become involved with psoriasis is the
    A. elbows
    B. knees
    C. antecubital fossa
    D. scalp
    E. back

740. Patients with acanthosis nigricans should be studied for
    A. a visceral carcinoma
    B. lymphoma
    C. diabetes mellitus
    D. sarcoidosis
    E. an allergy

266 / Diseases of the Skin

741. Treatment of acute contact dermatitis during the bullous, oozing stage should include
    A. bland compresses and baths
    B. corticosteroid ointments
    C. topical anesthetics
    D. systemic antibiotics
    E. antihistamines

742. Characteristic of ringworm fungi as compared with other fungi is their
    A. ability to digest and hydrolyze keratin
    B. high degree of contagiousness
    C. ability to invade the dermis
    D. sensitivity to penicillin
    E. ability to spread to other organs

743. Verrucae (warts)
    A. are viral in etiology
    B. may be premalignant lesions
    C. are found mainly in patients with a lymphoma
    D. are contagious in children only
    E. may be treated with griseofulvin

744. For skin disease to be considered occupational, the history should reveal all of the following EXCEPT
    A. other workmen affected
    B. no dermatitis preceding occupation
    C. worsening eruption during weekend
    D. list of chemicals contacted
    E. reappearance on return to work

745. Following the appearance of the primary chancre, the serologic test for syphilis may remain negative for a period not longer than
    A. one week
    B. two weeks
    C. one month
    D. three months
    E. six months

Diseases of the Skin / 267

746. Skin manifestations associated with chronic ulcerative colitis include all of the following EXCEPT
   A. maculopapular eruptions
   B. erythema nodosum
   C. pyoderma gangrenosum
   D. erythema multiforme
   E. necrobiosis lipoidica

747. Mycosis fungoides is best described as a
   A. fungal infection of the epidermis
   B. benign skin lesion
   C. cutaneous lymphoma
   D. dermatitis
   E. form of eczema

748. Rhinophyma is a complication of
   A. acne vulgaris
   B. pemphigus
   C. acne rosacea
   D. psoriasis
   E. seborrheic dermatitis

749. Vitiligo is characterized by the finding of areas of depigmentation of the skin. It is further characterized by
   A. the frequent finding of an underlying neoplastic disorder
   B. multiple pituitary deficiencies
   C. being a disorder of unknown etiology in most instances and being resistant to therapy
   D. its good response to ultraviolet therapy
   E. none of the above

750. von Recklinghausen's disease is characterized by all of the following EXCEPT
   A. areas of skin pigmentation
   B. pedunculated skin tumors
   C. multiple neural tumors
   D. tumors most frequently appearing during puberty
   E. viral etiology

DIRECTIONS: Each set of lettered headings below is followed by a list of numbered words or phrases. For each numbered word or phrase select

- **A** if the item is associated with (A) *only,*
- **B** if the item is associated with (B) *only,*
- **C** if the item is associated with *both* (A) *and* (B),
- **D** if the item is associated with *neither* (A) *nor* (B).

    A. Erythema multiforme (EM)
    B. Pemphigus
    C. Both
    D. Neither

751. Fatal in many instances, especially if untreated

752. Sharply demarcated macular lesion with a tendency to develop "target" lesions

753. Involvement of mucous membranes

754. Responds very well to sulfadiazine

755. Corticosteroids are the treatment of choice

    A. Psoriasis
    B. Seborrheic dermatitis
    C. Both
    D. Neither

756. Tendency to greasy skin

757. Exposure to sunlight is of therapeutic value

758. May be associated with rheumatoid arthritis

759. Frequent involvement of fingernails

760. High incidence of gastric neoplasia

   A. Squamous cell carcinoma of the skin
   B. Basal cell carcinoma of the skin
   C. Both
   D. Neither

761. Does not metastasize beyond the skin

762. May be caused by excessive exposure to sunlight

763. May be treated with x-ray therapy

764. Keratin pearls are seen pathologically

765. May develop in long-standing scars

   A. Scleroderma
   B. Dermatomyositis
   C. Both
   D. Neither

766. Heliotrope erythema

767. Mucous membrane involvement

768. Ulceration of the fingertips

769. Association with visceral disease

770. Renal disease

270 / Diseases of the Skin

DIRECTIONS: For each of the questions or incomplete statements below, **one** or **more** of the answers or completions given is correct. Select

    A if only *1, 2 and 3* are correct,
    B if only *1 and 3* are correct,
    C if only *2 and 4* are correct,
    D if only *4* is correct,
    E if *all* are correct.

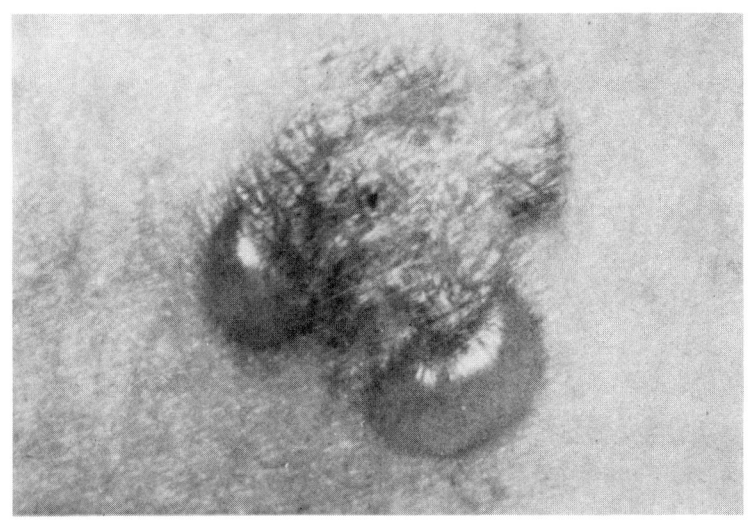

Figure 11.1

771. The skin lesion pictured in Figure 11.1 suggests a diagnosis of
 1. pemphigus vulgaris
 2. acanthosis nigricans
 3. pemphigoid
 4. herpes zoster

Diseases of the Skin / 271

772. Which of the following is characteristic of neurofibromatosis?
    1. Dominant inheritance
    2. Subcutaneous nodules along nerve sheaths
    3. Association with pheochromocytoma
    4. Pigmentary abnormalities

773. Benefit to patients with severe acne is usually obtained with
    1. dietary controls
    2. radiotherapy
    3. ultraviolet light
    4. low-dose antimicrobials

774. Which of the following is characteristic of Sezary's syndrome?
    1. Exfoliative erythroderma
    2. Folded cerebriform nuclei
    3. T-cell markers
    4. Responsiveness to cyclophosphamide

775. Which of the following features indicates a more negative prognosis for patients with malignant melanoma?
    1. Female sex
    2. Location on the leg
    3. Dark pigmentation of the lesion
    4. Nodularity of the lesion

11. Diseases of the Skin
   Answers and Comments

733. A. Koebner's phenomenon is typically seen in psoriasis. The kind of injury eliciting the phenomenon is usually mechanical, but ultraviolet light or allergic damage to the skin may be provocative. **(REF. 5, p. 234)**

734. A. Kaposi's sarcoma often manifests as multiple blue dermal plaques. Lesions have two prominent features: accumulation of spindle cells and presence of vascular elements. **(REF. 5, p. 745)**

735. B. Psoriasis does not present a progression of lesions unless therapy is applied. Lesions vary in size and configuration from patient to patient and in the same patient, from time to time. **(REF. 5, pp. 236–237)**

736. E. In dermatomyositis, the dermatitis may be the most striking feature of the illness or so minor as to be easily overlooked. **(REF. 5, p. 1300)**

737. D. A change of environment is among the best treatments for atopic dermatitis. The patient should be kept in as dust-free an environment as possible and should not wear rough garments. **(REF. 5, p. 526)**

738. B. This tumor as a rule occurs on exposed, hairy skin. It grows rapidly but involutes slowly, occasionally up to one year. **(REF. 5, p. 385)**

739. C. The antecubital fossa is the area least likely to be involved with psoriasis. The mucosal integuments are almost always free of lesions, presumably because cell kinetics are hyperactive normally. **(REF. 5, p. 238)**

740. A. Patients with acanthosis nigricans should be studied for a visceral carcinoma. Other dermatoses associated with malignancy include dermatomyositis, flushing, acquired ichthyosis, and thrombophlebitis migrans. **(REF.** 5, p. 1198)

741. A. Ointments are not used, but wet dressings are applied several times a day, using Burow's solution or boric acid, and baths are also included in the treatment. **(REF.** 5, p. 511)

742. A. The ability to digest and hydrolyze keratin is characteristic of ringworm fungi. Since dermatophytes fluoresce, an ultraviolet light with a Wood's filter may be used to identify infected hair. **(REF.** 5, p. 1522)

743. A. Verrucae are viral in etiology. The human papilloma virus is a DNA-containing virus of the papovirus group that includes animal tumor viruses. **(REF.** 5, p. 1631)

744. C. The history should not reveal worsening eruption during the weekend. Allergy, acne, diabetes, psoriasis, xeroderma, or seborrheic dermatitis may all be mistaken for occupational disorders. **(REF.** 5, p. 1010)

745. C. The STS may remain negative for a period not longer than one month after the appearance of the primary chancre. The STS usually becomes positive about one week after the chancre appears. With therapy the chancre heals in a week. **(REF.** 5, p. 1686)

746. E. Skin manifestations do not include necrobiosis lipoidica. Unlike the arthritis of ulcerative colitis, the dermatologic lesions respond to therapy to control the bowel disease. **(REF.** 5, pp. 1198–1199)

747. C. Mycosis fungoides is best described as a cutaneous lymphoma. Lesions may remain confined to the skin for years, and internal organ involvement occurs when the disease advances into late stages. **(REF.** 5, p. 750)

748. C. Rhinophyma is a complication of acne rosacea. It can be treated surgically by shaving off the excessive tissue with a scalpel, but regrowth occurs in time. **(REF.** 5, p. 454)

749. C. Vitiligo is ordinarily asymptomatic, but pruritus or burning may occur after exposure to sunlight. It is also characterized by being of unknown etiology in most instances and being resistant to therapy. **(REF. 5, p. 582)**

750. E. The disease is the result of the action of an abnormal gene of unknown location in the karyotype. **(REF. 5, p. 1217)**

751. B. Pemphigus is fatal in many instances, especially if untreated. Glucocorticoid administration is the mainstay of treatment; antibiotics may be required for secondary infection. **(REF. 5, pp. 295–302, 310–316)**

752. A. In erythema multiforme, vivid red blots appear suddenly in symmetrical distribution, favoring the extensor surfaces and distal limbs. **(REF. 5, pp. 295–302, 310–316)**

753. C. The mucous membranes are involved in both conditions. Oral lesions often occur in EM, leading first to blisters and then to erosions of the cheeks, gums, and tongue. **(REF. 5, pp. 295–302, 310–316)**

754. D. Neither condition responds to sulfadiazine. Oral antihistamines may hasten recovery in erythema multiforme. **(REF. 5, pp. 295–302, 310–316)**

755. B. Corticosteroids are the treatment of choice for pemphigus. Methotrexate may be used in patients with pemphigus in the early, localized stage of the disease. **(REF. 5, pp. 295–302, 310–316).**

756. B. Seborrheic dermatitis begins as a fine, branny scaling of the scalp and may involve the forehead, ears, neck, and face. It also produces a tendency to greasy skin. **(REF. 5, pp. 233–247, 803–807)**

757. C. Exposure to sunlight is of therapeutic value to both. Topical corticosteroids are active in seborrhea; but in psoriasis, ultraviolet light often works, especially from natural sunlight. **(REF. 5, pp. 233–247, 803–807)**

758. A. Psoriasis may be associated wtih rheumatoid arthritis. Involvement of the joints occurs in relatively few cases but can become a major disabling event. (**REF.** 5, pp. 233-247, 803-807)

759. A. Punctate pitting of the nail plate is characteristic but not diagnostic of psoriasis. (**REF.** 5, pp. 233-247, 803-807)

760. D. Neither is associated with a high incidence of gastric neoplasia. Conditions associated with underlying malignancy include dermatomyositis, acanthosis nigricans, and migratory thrombophlebitis. (**REF.** 5, pp. 233-247, 803-807)

761. B. Basal cell tumors have a substantial capacity for local destruction but metastasize very rarely. (**REF.** 5, pp. 362-383)

762. C. Sunlight is only one of many factors causing both, since carcinomas frequently appear in areas not maximally irradiated. (**REF.** 5, pp. 362-383)

763. C. In both carcinomas, early detection may lead to cure by surgical removal, but radiotherapy may be curative if used in high dosage. (**REF.** 5, pp. 362-383)

764. A. Invasive squamous cell carcinoma consists of malignant epidermal cells extending beyond the dermoepidermal junction. (**REF.** 5, pp. 362-383)

765. A. In squamous cell carcinoma of the skin, other early lesions include solar keratoses, cutaneous horns, arsenical keratoses, and Bowen's disease. (**REF.** 5, pp. 362-383)

766. B. This purplish red discoloration of the upper eyelids is almost diagnostic of dermatomyositis when seen. (**REF.** 5, pp. 1298-1313)

767. B. There is mucous membrane involvement in dermatomyositis. Papules and shallow ulcers occur in 10% to 20% of patients and may be associated with leukoplakia. (**REF.** 5, pp. 1298-1313)

276 / Diseases of the Skin

768. A. Scleroderma may be preceded by Raynaud's phenomenon or by chronic nonpitting edema of the fingers. **(REF. 5, pp. 1298-1313)**

769. C. Dermatomyositis may indicate an underlying malignancy, and scleroderma may involve the esophagus or the lungs. **(REF. 5, pp. 1298-1313)**

770. C. Acute renal failure from myoglobin may occur in dermatomyositis, and abrupt renal failure with hypertension is common in scleroderma. **(REF. 5, pp. 1298-1313)**

771. B. Pemphigus is characterized histologically by acantholysis, whereas pemphigoid causes bullae without acantholysis. **(REF. 1, pp. 2288, 2289)**

772. E. Neurofibromatosis is associated with systemic manifestations in the nervous system, bone, soft tissues, and skin. About 90% of patients have pigmentary abnormalities. **(REF. 1, p. 2279)**

773. D. Tetracyclines are commonly used in the treatment of acne but may be associated with risk of dental discoloration or photosensitivity. **(REF. 1, p. 2264)**

774. A. Sezary's syndrome resembles mycosis fungoides in many respects but does not respond well to chemotherapy with alkylating agents or to electron beam therapy. **(REF. 1, p. 2293)**

775. D. Nodular melanoma is invasive from the start. Women do better than men; trunk lesions and depigmented lesions carry a worse prognosis. **(REF. 1, p. 2294)**

12. Legal Medicine

DIRECTIONS: Each of the questions or incomplete statements below is followed by five suggested answers or completions. Select the **one** that is **best** in each case.

776. All of the following will probably constitute a coroner's case EXCEPT
    A. deaths associated with violence
    B. deaths in a chronic hospital
    C. cremation of a body before pronouncement
    D. nonattendance by a physician
    E. moving a body out of state

777. Even though soft tissue is destroyed prior to postmortem, it is usually possible to distinguish males from females by
    A. skeletal structure
    B. x-ray of the dentition
    C. length of the long bones
    D. joint degeneration
    E. closure of epiphyses

778. To establish time of death during the first 24 hours, assume a rate of cooling in average temperatures of
    A. 2°C per minute
    B. 10°C per hour
    C. 10°C per minute
    D. 2°C per hour
    E. 10°C per day

278 / Legal Medicine

779. In seeking evidence to document rape, if more than six hours have elapsed, the most likely specimen for detecting intact spermatozoa is
   A. vaginal aspirates
   B. seminal fluid dried on clothing or skin
   C. vulvar aspirates
   D. rectal aspirates
   E. oral aspirates

780. A physician called upon to treat a victim of the battered child syndrome should
   A. respect the physician-patient privilege
   B. respect the husband-wife privilege
   C. admonish the parents severely
   D. refuse to admonish the parents
   E. notify the hospital administrator or the police

781. Obtaining a written consent form rather than an oral consent has which of the following advantages?
   A. Exclusions may aid a patient's lawsuit
   B. Physician-patient rapport is improved
   C. Proof is better that informed consent was obtained
   D. It is administratively easier to accomplish
   E. It is generally the physician's preference

782. A physician is generally prohibited from signing a death certificate in cases that involve
   A. infectious disease
   B. suicide
   C. platelet emboli
   D. epilepsy
   E. venereal disease

DIRECTIONS: The group of questions below consists of five lettered headings followed by a list of numbered words, phrases or statements. For **each** numbered word, phrase or statement, select the **one** lettered heading that is most closely associated with it. Each lettered heading may be selected once, more than once, or not at all.

- A. Abrasion
- B. Contusion
- C. Laceration
- D. Blunt trauma
- E. Penetrating wounds

783. Displacement of the epidermis by friction

784. The severity of the injury cannot be estimated by the size of the cutaneous defect

785. Internal organs may be lacerated without damage to the surface of the body

786. Extravasated blood diffusely distributed through the tissue spaces

787. Most commonly seen in areas where the skin is stretched over bony eminences

280 / Legal Medicine

DIRECTIONS: For each of the questions or incomplete statements below, **one** or **more** of the answers or completions given is correct. Select

    A if only *1, 2 and 3* are correct,
    B if only *1 and 3* are correct,
    C if only *2 and 4* are corect,
    D if only *4* is correct,
    E if *all* are correct.

788. In arranging artificial insemination, which of the following points should be covered in the agreement with the parties?
    1. The wife should consent in writing
    2. Written consent of the donor's wife should be obtained
    3. The physician should have permission to select the donor
    4. The donor should consent in writing

789. Consent for surgery may be invalid in cases in which
    1. the act consented to is unlawful
    2. it is not an informed consent
    3. it was obtained by misinterpretation
    4. a parent signs for a child

790. In order to comply with regulations concerning narcotics prescriptions, every practicing physician should
    1. register with the Bureau of Narcotics every five years
    2. utilize a federal narcotics order form to secure an office supply
    3. order narcotics by telephone only if he knows the pharmacist
    4. list his registry number on every prescription

791. Which of the following criteria are necessary for the diagnosis of "brain death"?
    1. No response to external stimuli
    2. Only reflex breathing
    3. A flat isoelectric electroencephalogram
    4. No reflexes for a four-hour period

792. If a patient's fractured arm is set poorly but the patient refuses to allow the physician to reset the arm, liability for negligence rests with
    1. the patient
    2. the hospital
    3. the patient's next of kin
    4. the physician

793. Damages awarded in a judicial proceeding for any injury may be classified as
    1. inordinate
    2. nominal
    3. retroactive
    4. punitive

794. The legal judgment of sanity or insanity is relevant to cases of
    1. impaired driving
    2. capability to make a will
    3. ownership of property
    4. competence to testify

795. Revocation of the license to practice medicine commonly occurs on which of the following grounds?
    1. Conviction of a felony
    2. Drug addiction
    3. Professional liability
    4. Practicing chiropractic

Directions Summarized

A	B	C	D	E
1,2,3 only	1,3 only	2,4 only	4 only	All are correct

796. In drawing up a medical partnership, a sound agreement should include
    1. profit and loss sharing
    2. partner's negligence
    3. retirement or death
    4. additional partners

797. Statutes of limitation, providing periods of time during which legal action must be instituted, may be delayed in onset by the
    1. fraudulent concealment of the wrongful act
    2. death of the patient
    3. impossibility of detection
    4. request of the patient's lawyer

798. Investigation of body fluid stains may include which of the following?
    1. Isoenzyme phenotypes analysis
    2. ABH substance detection
    3. Sex chromatin determinations
    4. Species origin determination

799. When collecting specimens for analysis of possible poisons, it is best to save
    1. the most suspicious items
    2. vomitus, if present
    3. items using washed containers
    4. bowel contents, if available

800. Blunt injuries may create medicolegal problems because
   1. there is no visible wound
   2. the injuries are usually minor
   3. there may be a long time-lapse
   4. surgery is relatively contraindicated

12. Legal Medicine
Answers and Comments

776. B. Between 15% and 20% of all deaths that occur in the United States are related to violence, or to unexplained or unexpected causes. Deaths in a chronic hospital will not constitute a coroner's case. **(REF. 3, p. 6)**

777. A. In the case of mutilated or decomposed bodies or fragments, evidence establishing the sex of the dead person may be the first step in identity and can probably be determined by skeletal stucture. **(REF. 3, p. 14)**

778. D. Assume a rate of cooling in average temperatures of 2°C per hour. Post-mortem heat loss is accelerated in cold environments and by passage of air currents over the body or by low humidity. **(REF. 3, p. 16)**

779. B. The most likely specimen is seminal fluid dried on clothing or skin. Ordinarily, spermatozoa have either migrated out of the vagina or have disintegrated after a lapse of 6 to 12 hours. **(REF. 3, p. 72)**

780. E. The report to the hospital administrator or the police is to be made immediately by telephone and to be followed thereafter in writing. **(REF. 3, p. 75)**

781. C. Written consent is better proof that informed consent was obtained. Other advantages are that it provides a written checklist and a deterrent to a malpractice lawsuit. Disadvantages include weakening of physician rapport with patient. **(REF. 3, p. 215)**

782. B. A death certificate should not be signed if there is any violent or suspicious death whether homicidal, suicidal, or accidental. **(REF. 3, pp. 7–8)**

783. A. An abrasion displaces the epidermis by friction. The location and character of an abrasion may help to establish the circumstances in which more severe injuries were sustained. **(REF. 3, p. 31)**

784. E. In penetrating wounds, the severity of the injury cannot be estimated by the size of the cutaneous defect. Firearm injuries comprise the majority of penetrating wounds other than stab wounds. **(REF. 3, p. 33)**

785. D. The internal structures most frequently damaged include bones, ligaments, meningeal vessels, the brain, and the spinal cord. In blunt trauma, internal organs may be lacerated without damage to the surface of the body. **(REF. 3, p. 32)**

786. B. In contusions, extravasated blood is diffusely distributed through the tissue spaces. Multiple contusions from minor trauma are often encountered in alcoholic females and may lend false importance to the role of physical violence. **(REF. 3, p. 31)**

787. C. Lacerations are most commonly seen in areas where the skin is stretched over bony eminences. The skin on the side of the wound opposite to the direction of motion is usually undermined for a variable distance. **(REF. 3, p. 32)**

788. E. All of the listed points should be covered. The physician should also establish to his own satisfaction that, from the medical point of view, the husband is sterile. **(REF. 3, p. 187)**

789. A. Consent should be explained to the patient in understandable, nontechnical terms. Authority may come from a legally appointed guardian, as well as from a parent signing for a child. **(REF. 3, p. 213)**

790. C. Telephone orders for narcotics are prohibited whether a prescription covering such orders is subsequently received or not. The physician should use a federal narcotics order form to secure an office supply, and he should list his registry number on every prescription. **(REF. 3, p. 281)**

791. B. No response to external stimuli and a flat isoelectric electroencephalogram are necessary for the diagnosis of "brain death." In addition, signs must be absent for 24 hours, the patient must not be on sedatives, and the temperature should be over 90° F. **(REF. 3, p. 293)**

792. D. A patient's negligence is not "contributory" if it merely aggravates an injury caused by the doctor's negligence. Liability for negligence rests with the physician. **(REF. 3, p. 196)**

793. C. The three kinds of damages awarded may be nominal, compensatory or actual, and punitive or exemplary. **(REF. 3, p. 198)**

794. C. Legal judgment is relevant to cases of capability to make a will and competence to testify. There is no mental disease called "insanity." Insanity is a legal term for certain people who exhibit particular symptoms of mental disease. **(REF. 3, p. 167)**

795. A. Revocation commonly occurs on the grounds of conviction of a felony, drug addiction, and professional liability. Other grounds for revocation include gross indecency, false advertising, fraud in application, and alcoholism. **(REF. 3, p. 223)**

796. E. A sound agreement should include all of the items listed. Other clauses on the agreement should include capital contributions, expenses, vacations, withdrawal, and expulsions. **(REF. 3, p. 204)**

797. B. They may be delayed in onset by the fraudulent concealment of the wrongful act and by the impossibility of detection. The statutory period is delayed also in the case of a minor until the patient attains the age of majority. **(REF. 3, p. 315)**

798. E. Body fluids can be studied also from the point of view of MN, Lewis, Secretor status, immunoglobulin isotypes, and time-lapse since formation of the stain. **(REF.** 3, pp. 145-157)

799. C. It is best to save anything and everything even though not apparently suspicious. Washed containers may be contaminated even if washed thoroughly, so that it is best to use clean plastic bags. **(REF.** 3, pp. 118-119)

800. B. In most blunt injuries, signs and symptoms appear rapidly, but traumatically induced cranial or abdominal injury may not manifest for several hours. **(REF.** 3, p. 40)

References

1. Wyngaarden, J.B., Smith, L.H.: *Cecil Textbook of Medicine,* 16th Ed., Philadelphia, W.B. Saunders Co., 1982.

2. Isselbacher, K.J., et al.: *Harrison's Principles of Internal Medicine,* 9th Ed., New York, McGraw-Hill Book Co., 1980.

3. Hirsch, C.S., Morris, R.C., Moritz, A.R.: *Handbook of Legal Medicine,* 5th Ed., St. Louis, C.V. Mosby Co., 1979.

4. Wintrobe, M.M., et al.: *Clinical Hematology,* 8th Ed., Philadelphia, Lea and Febiger, 1981.

5. Fitzpatrick, T.B., et al.: *Dermatology in General Medicine,* 2nd Ed., New York, McGraw-Hill Book Co., 1979.

6. Merritt, H.H.: *A Textbook of Neurology,* 6th Ed., Philadelphia, Lea and Febiger, 1979.

7. Williams, R.H.: *Textbook of Endocrinology,* 6th Ed., Philadelphia, W.B. Saunders Co., 1981.

8. Gilman, A.G., Goodman, L.S., Gilman, A.: *The Pharmacological Basis of Therapeutics,* 6th Ed., New York, Macmillan Publishing Co., 1980.

9. Bondy, P.K., Rosenberg, L.E.: *Metabolic Control and Disease,* 8th Ed., Philadelphia, W.B. Saunders Co., 1980.

10. Hurst, J.W., et al.: *The Heart,* 5th Ed., New York, McGraw-Hill Book Co., 1982.

11. Stanbury, J.B., Wyngaarden, J.B., Fredrickson, D.S.: *The Metabolic Basis of Inherited Disease,* 4th Ed., New York, McGraw-Hill Book Co., 1978.

BOOKS OF RELATED INTEREST:

NATIONAL BOARDS EXAMINATION REVIEW
    Part One: Basic Sciences   #103 $26.50
    Part Two: Clinical Sciences   #101 $26.50

FLEX REVIEW   #158 $27.50

ECFMG/FMG EXAMINATION REVIEW
    Part One   #120 $16.95
    Part Two   #121 $16.95

FMG EXAMINATION REVIEW
    Volume 1: Basic Sciences   #124 $16.95
    Volume 2: Clinical Sciences   #125 $16.95

INTERNAL MEDICINE Specialty Board
Review, Seventh Edition   #303 $28.50

Use this coupon today to order the books listed above or those on the back cover!

MEDICAL EXAMINATION PUBLISHING CO., INC.
an Excerpta Medica company

3003 New Hyde Park Road
New Hyde Park, New York 11040

|IBP|

Please print your selection(s):

quantity code #   author   title   price

_____ @ _____
_____ @ _____
_____ @ _____

ALL PRICES SUBJECT TO CHANGE
☐ To save shipping and handling charges, my check is enclosed. (New York residents, please add sales tax.)

NAME _____
ADDRESS _____
CITY _____ STATE _____ ZIP _____
SIGNATURE _____

AVAILABLE AT BOOKSTORES OR BY USING THIS COUPON